THE PATCHWORK MOUSE

THE PATCHWORK MOUSE

joseph hixson

ANCHOR PRESS/DOUBLEDAY
GARDEN CITY, NEW YORK
1976

Grateful acknowledgment is made for permission to quote from the following:

"Science Denies Cancer Research Fraud," by Jane Brody, May 29, 1974. Copyright © 1974 by the New York Times Company. Reprinted by permission.

Speech by Dr. James Watson given at the dedication of the Seeley G. Mudd Biological Sciences Building at MIT, March 1975. Used by permission of Dr. James Watson.

The Journal of the American Medical Association, September 9, 1974, Vol. 229, No. 11 p. 1391. Copyright 1974 by the American Medical Association.

"The Sloan-Kettering Affair," J. H. Raaf and J. L. Ninnemann, *Science,* Vol. 185, p. 734, 30 August 1975. Copyright 1975 by the American Association for the Advancement of Science. Used by permission.

"Immunologic Modification: A Basic Survival Mechanism," B. B. Jacobs and D. D. Uphoff, *Science,* Vol. 185, p. 582–87, 16 August 1974. Copyright 1974 by the American Association for the Advancement of Science. Used by permission.

"The Sloan-Kettering Affair: A Story Without a Hero," Barbara J. Culliton, *Science,* Vol. 184, pp. 644–50, 10 May 1974. Copyright 1974 by the American Association for the Advancement of Science. Used by permission.

"The Sloan-Kettering Affair (II): An Uneasy Resolution," Barbara J. Culliton, *Science,* Vol. 184, pp. 1154–57, 14 June 1974. Copyright 1974 by the American Association for the Advancement of Science. Used by permission.

Library of Congress Cataloging in Publication Data

Hixson, Joseph R
 The patchwork mouse.

 Includes index.
  1. Cancer research—United States. 2. Summerlin,
William Talley, 1938– I. Title.
RC267.H58 616.9'94'0724
ISBN: 0-385-02852-0
Library of Congress Catalog Card Number 74-27583

This book is dedicated to the late Dr. DAVID KARNOFSKY, a gentleman who fought cancer as devotedly as anyone, who died of it bravely at home, and who kept his skepticism about progress against the disease always in the path of those in a hurry to see such advances.

JRH

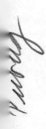

This book is dedicated to the late Dr. Lynn
Karvasky, a gentleman who fought cancer scientifically as best
he knew how and at times, ruthlessly, pitting desperate
allout progress against the line he always had in quiet choice or
fancy to his unjust adversary.

CONTENTS

PREFACE

The events narrated in this book cover about seven years in the immediate past and about half a century all told. A behind-the-scenes account of the politics of cancer research in the United States is susceptible to a number of approaches, both chronologically and as to focus. The version that follows is the result of considerable negotiation between me and my editor at Doubleday.

I hope that by the time the reader has reached the end of the book, he or she will have enough information to form an opinion about what is good and what is not so good in our current system of medical research as it pertains to cancer. If reader disagrees with author, why then, so much the better. He has obviously not been offered a pair of loaded dice.

Some critical remarks appear in the following pages having to do with cancer fund raising by individual institutions, the American Cancer Society and others. I would hope that readers would not infer anything improper, much less scandalous, in the way these agencies and facilities go about obtaining support. Those who run them must pay bills and the money must be raised to pay those bills. As in advertising for soap products and automobiles, there are entrepreneurs (agencies) in the medical fund-raising area whose writers, whether for posters, direct-mail pieces, or publicity handouts, often seek out the selling proposition in preference to the one that is strictly accurate. Usually such excessive claims are pruned down by the organization that is purchasing the service, but the temptation is always there to make things sound a little faster-moving than they really are. In reference to slogans, catch phrases, and so forth used in cancer campaigns, I mean no more than to urge vigilance on the part of the targets of these efforts, just as, in the Epilogue on news media, I urge viewers, readers, and listeners to take news of progress against cancer with a heavy dose of skepticism.

Among my thanks to many people who have given a lot of time in helping me to try to understand what has been going on and in looking at various drafts of the manuscript, I also have to regret that one of the principal figures in the book declined (on advice of counsel) to be interviewed about his side of the story. Then, too, there were several scientists who wished to offer extremely critical views so long as their names were omitted. Their anecdotes, which would certainly have enlivened the following pages, were rejected for reasons that should be easy to understand. The testimony of "Deep Throats" is clearly essential when the welfare of the Republic is at stake. In science reporting, however, we have had entirely too much unattributable gossip already, especially in the areas covered by this book. I didn't get into the topic of scientific courage, the guts to make your dissent public no matter how it affects your tenure and grants. But there's plenty to be said about that, too, another time.

THE PATCHWORK MOUSE

1

CREPES AND CHAMPAGNE

WHEN THE TWO young women came out onto Third
Avenue in Manhattan's East Seventies it was still pitch dark. On
the major avenues of New York, however, taxis are cruising for
fares at five o'clock in the morning. The driver who stopped to
pick up Manette Charny and Lana Hart probably didn't even
notice the bags they were carrying. And if he had known that the
two young secretaries were lugging warm crepes and jam and a
bottle of chilled champagne to one of the country's better known

cancer research laboratories for a predawn breakfast, the cabbie would likely have put that away with all his other mental jottings of the idiosyncrasies peculiar to the residents of the city's most fashionable section.

The ride was a short one, not more than half a mile, to the Kettering Laboratory on the north side of East Sixty-eighth Street just short of York Avenue. The driver would know that area as a major medical crossroads of Manhattan where the white, Gothic bulk of New York Hospital towers over the manicured grounds of Rockefeller University and where, across the street, workmen had only recently completed the new Memorial Hospital with its six hundred beds allotted to frightened patients with cancer.

The two secretaries went into the twelve-story building and took the elevator up to the sixth floor and the small suite of offices where their boss had spent the night on his cot. Dr. William Talley Summerlin, late of Minneapolis, had been in New York less than a year in March of 1974. But for a thirty-five-year-old dermatologist born in a small town in South Carolina and educated in Atlanta, Dr. Summerlin's arrival at the Memorial Sloan-Kettering Cancer Center marked an enormous increase in prestige and pay. As the new director of the Sloan-Kettering Institute, the research arm of the cancer center, Dr. Robert Alan Good had the power to elevate his protégés from the University of Minnesota to any level he wanted. In Dr. Summerlin's case, the move from Minneapolis meant appointment as chief of Memorial Hospital's cutaneous disease service and, in the institute, as a full member, the academic equivalent in university medical circles of full professor. Thus the tall, balding young skin specialist was the proprietor of two sets of offices and secretaries, together with a stable of nurses, technicians, and young postdoctoral fellows to support his experiments on the transplantation of skin and other organs.

He hoped these would prove that tissues that had been nurtured in a laboratory culture for several weeks could then be transplanted to genetically different animals without provoking rejection by the recipient's immune system. If successful, these findings would have important implications for organ transplantation and cancer therapy, which immunologists believe are closely related. Doctors have observed that the body's normal immune system acts as a barrier to cancer. Every year more than 350,000 Americans die of cancer. Yet the number of cases doctors see is now thought to make up only a small fraction of those that occur and are aborted by body defenses. Efforts such as Summerlin's in preventing rejection of transplanted organs could tell us why the body's immune system occasionally fails to act. Because of this time-consuming research, Summerlin's wife and the three young sons were accustomed to the doctor's absence at least two nights a week from their Darien, Connecticut, home.

When the young women came into their office adjoining the cubicle where their boss had spent the night, a postdoctoral research fellow and a technician were already there. Breakfast had to be early because Good liked to schedule meetings with members of his staff as the sun was coming up. This morning, Tuesday, March 26, Summerlin was on the calendar for 7 A.M.

Manette and Lana had almost abandoned the caper the night before. The idea of serving crepes and champagne for breakfast had come up when Summerlin had asked one of his technicians and one of his research fellows to come in very early so that they could help him change the dressings on some mice he wanted to take across the street to show Good the next morning. The animals bore patches of skin from other mice, patches that had been carefully nourished in laboratory glassware for several weeks after removal from their previous owners and before being sewed on the backs of their new hosts. Summerlin had made a kidding remark to the two assistants, offering to buy them breakfast after his meeting with the director of Sloan-Kettering to make up for their loss of sleep. That was when Manette had offered to make crepes for breakfast. Then, later, Lana had remembered the bottle of unopened champagne in her refrigerator, a gift that had been stored there awaiting an occasion. Summerlin's staff on the research side were a close-knit group who liked their boss and worked long hours for him. In addition, the breakfast offer came as a gesture of support for the doctor. Both women had sensed their boss's increasing anxiety of late, and

they were aware that relations between Summerlin and at least
two of the research fellows were unusually strained. One of them,
unable to reproduce his chief's test results, was about to publish
a report that would contradict everything Summerlin had been
telling the world for the past two years.

The two secretaries had worked late the night before, their
desks crowded with two others into the outer office between
their boss's sanctum and the room right off the hall that was used
by a couple of the research fellows. All three spaces were
typically laboratory, their cinder-block walls barely covered by
the institutional green paint. Across the hall were the actual
laboratories with their sinks and centrifuges, racks of clean
beakers and test tubes and the tall refrigerator and incubator
doors bearing crayoned warnings against meddling.

Five stories above, in Kettering's animal quarters, mice were
scurrying about in the darkness while neighboring rats and rabbits slept or crouched silently in their shiny metal bins, each
tagged with red or buff cards identifying their pedigree and
owner.

Around six, the champagne cork was popped, the wine poured
into small glasses, and the crepes smeared with jam. The party,
lasting only about twenty minutes, was later to be accorded
concern that might have better suited an all-night bacchanalia.

After breakfast, Summerlin and his helpers went on up to
the eleventh floor to select the best-looking grafted mice to be
shown to Good. Two of the animals chosen for the trip across
Sixty-eighth Street were albinos on whose backs skin cells from
black mice had been grafted. The dressings Summerlin pre-
ferred weren't bandages in the usual sense but fresh skin taken
from genetically identical mice and sewn over the graft. These
dressings had now to be removed so that Good might see how
well the grafts beneath were taking.

When the preparations had been completed, Summerlin took
the bin with a dozen of his best exhibits and set off for the
elevator bank and for Good's large office on the thirteenth floor
of the Howard Laboratory just under the penthouse in which the
director lived with his wife, Joanne. Manette and Lana went
back down to the sixth floor and rinsed out the glasses and

tidied up. Manette was going to class across the East River in Queens that morning, so she lay down on the doctor's cot and took a nap so as not to fall asleep in her biology course. When she got back from college in the afternoon, Summerlin wasn't around. And he didn't return before she left to go home at six. Manette thought that was a little strange.

Robert Good has shaved and pulled a white turtleneck shirt over his dark, tousled head at an hour when the swinging East Side singles bars have barely closed their doors. He has never wanted or needed more than about four or five hours of sleep a night. At 5:30 A.M., therefore, the director's rubbery features may be sagging a bit more than usual, but he is thoroughly alert and ready to bring his formidable intelligence to bear on medical and scientific matters, especially those in his chosen field of transplantation and tumor immunology.

As the director was leafing through the paper mound on his desk that March morning waiting for his protégé to appear, Summerlin was taking a little extra time in the elevator across the street. After pressing the black square numbered "1," he set the bin of mice upon the floor of the car. He then pulled two white mice from the container. While they wriggled and squeaked in protest, he inspected the sites of the black skin grafts. When grown in culture, such cells tend to lose their pigmentation, so the black-on-white patches appeared more a dirty gray than anything else. Impulsively, Summerlin took his felt-tipped pen out of the breast pocket of his white coat and applied it briefly to the grafted patches on the two white animals. The ink made them look darker. Then he replaced the mice in the bin and strode on out of the Kettering lobby.

The conference between Good and Summerlin was not an unusual event, but such sessions had become much rarer during the year in New York than they had been in Minneapolis. As director of the Sloan-Kettering Institute, Good had many more responsibilities than he had shouldered as a research professor, albeit one with a considerable empire, at the University of Minnesota. This plus Summerlin's expanded duties had been keeping the two men apart. But Good, fifteen years senior to the dermatologist, had been getting complaints about some of the work of the younger man, and they worried him. For two years Good had been telling eminent scientists, potential donors of funds, and every medical and science reporter who came near him that Summerlin's work in successfully transplanting cells after a period in tissue culture looked like a major immunologic breakthrough, if it could be confirmed.

While in his early thirties, at Stanford University in California, Summerlin had adopted a technique developed by a senior researcher there for growing skin cells in laboratory glassware. He had applied the method to the problem of transplantation rejection. Without conducting further animal tests, Summerlin had removed small bits of skin from one patient, cultured it in the special nutrient broth formulated by his colleague, a scientist but not a physician, and then, after four or five weeks, had transferred the cells from their flask to another patient. The recipient, who should have sloughed off the donated cells from an unrelated stranger had, Summerlin reported, adopted them as his own. This had been accomplished, he said, without the aid of any drugs or serums to suppress the immune reaction that should promptly have destroyed the graft.

The report of this accomplishment in four separate skin exchanges—and skin is, if anything, more subject to graft rejection than kidney or heart or liver or pancreas—had brought their innovator considerable attention in medical circles. Good's imagination, too, was stimulated by the notion that organ culture intervening between excision and transplantation might help solve one of the most vexing problems of modern surgery. It might also help provide clues in cancer research. Defense against cancer is, together with transplant rejection, one of the many functions carried out by the immune system. While Good was not a surgeon, he was a research professor at the University of Minnesota with several millions of dollars in grants at his disposal to fund his sizable group of scientists. And his varied accomplishments in the field of transplantation immunity caused his name to come up whenever potential Nobel prize recipients were discussed.

Once Summerlin had deserted Stanford to join Good at Minneapolis, he quickly learned that four human skin grafts and an engaging charm had nothing to do with what Good refers to reverently as "the method of science." The young skin specialist was quickly set to learning his immunologic lessons, getting acquainted with mouse genetic strains between which transplants would be more or less difficult, and then starting the grinding labor of exchanging skin between them to see whether his cell-culture technique could produce carefully controlled and documented successes when none would have been expected.

Summerlin had worked pretty much alone in Minneapolis, with Good near at hand, of course, to lend advice and criticism and encouragement. Then the financiers who run the Memorial Sloan-Kettering Cancer Center had, after a year's search, fastened upon Good as the man to replace the previous Sloan-Kettering director, Dr. Frank Horsfall, who had succumbed to pancreatic cancer early in 1971. Good had accepted, and the move to New York with a staff of fifty researchers, including Summerlin, had occupied much of the new director's time in the fall of 1972. It was precisely during this period that his newest protégé was broadening his claims to include other animals besides mice and organs other than skin (the body's largest organ). Good was not just bringing Summerlin with him. He was appointing him—or having him appointed—to the rank of full professor. Summerlin was then thirty-four.

He had been given plenty to do once he got to New York. He was to run the dermatology clinic, a new entity at Sloan-Kettering's sister institution, Memorial Hospital for Cancer and Allied Diseases. He was also expected to supervise the work of half a dozen postdoctoral fellows, who would further check the transplantation claims he had made and extend the immunologic research. This became increasingly important as reports filtered in to Good that scientists in other renowned research laboratories were having trouble corroborating the Summerlin data.

By March of 1974 Summerlin was frequently sleeping in his small office in the Kettering lab. He was to claim later that he was overworked. Others were to state that he was underorganized. In any case, reports coming in from around the world and also from the postdoctoral fellows at Sloan-Kettering were disturbing to Good. Staff members and others had been complaining about the dermatologist's sloppy habits—appointments broken, letters unanswered, and written reports containing obvious errors in arithmetic. That winter some of the research fellows were telling the director that they could not duplicate the animal grafting results that Summerlin was still saying confirmed his human experiments at Stanford.

At issue on that March morning in 1974 after a night spent on his cot was Summerlin's answer to the impending publication of one of his juniors reporting total failure to prolong the survival of any mouse skin grafts by growing the cells in culture first. If such a report were to be submitted to a professional journal, it would have to bear Summerlin's name as chief of the laboratory in which the tests had been made.

Robert Good can speak persuasively and without notes for an hour and more, his diagrams and slides flashing on and off a screen. The performance is never corny, theatrical, or evangelistic.

If Good desires attention, he gets it. There is no legato, there are no pregnant pauses, just a rush of information deftly tinted with the urgency of understanding pathologic processes in order to get at them. No scientist, tycoon, or government bureaucrat with or without a Ph.D. stands a chance of flustering Good or throwing his gentle bulk off balance. A swimmer might as well try to capsize a tugboat.

Oddly, Good didn't pay any attention to the animals Summerlin had brought over from the Kettering Laboratory that morning. Preoccupied with the apparently wobbly scientific pagoda Summerlin had erected, the director barely accorded the animals a glance. It would have taken only a second or two for Good's practiced eye to have spotted the doctored skin. Pathologists are the closest thing medicine has to an intellectual elite, and at Minnesota Robert Good had had the rank of professor both in pathology and pediatrics.

The meeting lasted forty-five minutes. Afterward, Summerlin returned to the Kettering Laboratory. He could have obliterated his inking of the mouse skins with a quick scrub of the mice using a ball of cotton soaked in a little alcohol. But the physician went up to the eleventh floor and turned the binful of mice over to James Martin, the laboratory assistant entrusted with the task of restoring the animals to their properly tagged containers. Engaged in this task, a few moments later, Martin noticed what the director had not. Two of his charges looked different. They had black patches that he had not seen before. It was Martin, not Summerlin, who performed the alcohol scrub and who, in astonishment, told a coworker and research technician, William Walter, of the coloring job. Walter, seeking a superior, first found a visiting research fellow from Ireland, Dr. Geoffrey O'Neill. O'Neill had only been at the institute for a couple of months and sought a more experienced hand in which to drop his incredible news. He went to Dr. John Raaf, another postdoctoral fellow, down from the Department of Surgery at Boston's Massachusetts General Hospital. O'Neill sensed that the visiting doctor from Boston, although youthful, had the background and experience to know what to do. Raaf did. He went straight across the street to seek out Good. When one of the executive secretaries on 13 Howard told him Good was in the center's monthly board meeting, Raaf insisted she get him out. Good came out to find a very agitated young man who blurted out the story. Good later recalled, "I came out of the meeting with Dr. Old [Lloyd J. Old, an eminent young Sloan-Kettering immunologic researcher serving as Good's deputy director of the Institute] and Dr. Raaf told us that Dr. Summerlin had blackened the skins of some white mice that he had shown me that morning. This was of such major concern because the big question Summerlin had always been asked was could he put the C57 black skin on the white A strain. So when Dr. Raaf told me this, I excused myself from the board meeting in the hospital and went straight upstairs to my office and called Dr. Summerlin and told him to come over and bring the mice that he had showed me in the morning. He came over about noontime, and Dr. Old was with me, and he said he couldn't bring the mice with him because he had just put on physiological dressings [skin from the same strain as the recipient mice that was laid on top of the grafts]. He didn't come in shamefaced and trying to tell me something. He breezed in in his usual way.

"I asked him to sit down and I said, 'Bill, it's come to my attention that you painted the skins black on some of the mice you showed me this morning to make them look as though they'd had successful transplants.' And at that point, in the presence of Dr. Old, he admitted having done that. And I said, "You know the implications of this?' This was the first time that I really doubted Summerlin's veracity. There had been plenty of problems about the science, but this was the first time I had doubted Summerlin's honesty. Right then, a kaleidoscope of questions went through my mind about the mice with guinea-pig skin grafts that had been prolonged and the white skin on the brown mice and the white skin on the black mice and the black skin on the white mice that he had showed us before, all the grafts he had presented to us in the past. I realized that no matter how closely I could have watched, I could have been fooled. And I could think of all the ways."

Good went on, "Right then, I said to him that we would have to suspend him temporarily while we looked into it. I don't remember whether it was then or later in a note to him I indicated that I would make a temporary suspension of two weeks while we looked at the issue and decided what was to be done."

Sometime earlier in the morning—Summerlin has said that it was around ten-thirty—Summerlin called the director's office but could not get through to him in the board meeting.

The gods who watch over pride and arrogance sometimes employ lesser mortals to be their tragic engines. They had chosen cannily in James Martin, animal caretaker. Whether the absurd gesture of touching up the mice had been a call for help from an overstressed psyche, as Summerlin was later to imply, or a sudden challenge to a mentor who seemed to the young researcher to have become a distant and hostile tormentor, it seems reasonable to assume that, had he detected the obvious painting himself, Good might have counseled rest and relaxation for his overwrought colleague. But the news had come through sources that already had reason to focus suspicion on Summerlin, and Good knew that his stance must be one of rigid adherence to the code that binds all scientists together.

Under this code, any misrepresentation of an experiment would jeopardize the offender's career unless and until a committee of his peers has investigated the matter and found him blameless. Bill Summerlin was sent home to Darien pending the formation of such a committee and a report of its findings and verdict.

2

MASTER ANd ApprENTICE

THE DECISION TO expose his protégé to a searching scientific inquiry, with all the ugly publicity attendant upon that process, did not please Dr. Good. Yet he offered this as a solution that afternoon to his superior, Dr. Lewis Thomas, president of the cancer center, and to Dr. Edward J. Beattie, Jr., chief medical officer of Memorial Hospital. When they promptly accepted the plan and ratified Summerlin's suspension, Good knew he was in for months of sniping from senior scientists at the institute,

whose comfortable domains he was in the process of dismembering, and from some distinguished colleagues around the nation
who had long thought the fifty-one-year-old director pushy and
self-aggrandizing.

A year before, a couple of them had spoken out anonymously
to an associate editor of *Time* magazine, Peter Stoler, when
Good's photograph adorned the magazine's cover with the caption TOWARD CONTROL OF CANCER. In his article, Stoler had attributed the snide comments he had garnered to jealousy of
Good's "ability to attract research funds and keep his name
before the public." The *Time* cover, itself, was a mark of distinc-
at it. The last person accorded this accolade for medical reasons
had been heart-transplanter Dr. Christiaan Barnard more than
tion or evidence of this proclivity, depending on how you looked
five years before. And no fires of resentment ever smoldered
more acridly in the spleens of America's top surgeons than did
those that griped their bellies when they saw the flamboyant
South African on *Time*'s cover.

However, Good had not earned his fame as a cancer researcher,
but as an immunologist, devoted to pursuing the age-old riddle
of how animals, including man, tell self from non-self. Yet, in the
last two decades, understanding cancer had become more and
more dependent upon this critical distinction.

Good was born to educators in Crosby, Minnesota, in 1922, the
second of four sons. His father, a high school principal, contracted cancer when Good was five and died that same year. The
boy, watching his father's doctor in awe, decided then and there
to enter medicine. After the father's death, Good's mother went
back to teaching school amid the hard times of the thirties. Good
worked as a section hand on the railroad and took other odd jobs
to help keep bread on the family table. Eventually he entered
the University of Minnesota.

Graduating in 1944 with a B.A. in zoology, he came to the attention of a well-to-do businessman who offered support for his
years at Minnesota's medical school. At this point, his career
almost ended with a virus infection that Good now believes was
not poliomyelitis as it was then diagnosed. He thinks it was
another agent, a virus that also attacks the nervous system but

more symmetrically and with less permanent damage, and whose symptoms are denoted by the names of the French doctors who first described them, Guillain-Barré. Partially paralyzed, Good added a rigorous exercise schedule to his freshman medical school grind and emerged from the experience with a limp from ankle weakness that has added yet another characteristic feature to his attire, basketball sneakers. (A rather starchy official of the Memorial Sloan-Kettering Center was startled to learn from a subordinate that the institute's director-designate had been seen in one of the fancier of the First Avenue restaurants lunching in his turtleneck and sneakers. Good's comment: "I've never been convinced that a necktie has any real function except to get in the way.")

At the end of his first year in medical school Good went to the dean, Dr. Harold Diehl (later to become a scientific vice president of the American Cancer Society) to ask that he be allowed to go for his Ph.D. in anatomy in addition to his regular medical studies. Diehl denied the request instantly. Did Mr. Good understand the rigors of the sophomore medical course? The thing was ridiculous on the face of it. Forty-two credits in one term? Preposterous. Good was forced to make a concession to get his way. Any mark below a B, and he would drop the anatomy doctorate courses. A grudging acquiescence from Dean Diehl. That first term Good received an A in forty of the credits and a B in the other two.

In his last two years of medical school his anatomy studies steered Good to his abiding interest in the lymph-gland immunologic system. His Ph.D. minor in microbiology, and perhaps his brush with paralysis, produced a strong curiosity about viruses and their behavior. (Good's first published scientific paper in 1945 involved the ways in which herpes viruses either take over their cellular hosts and destroy them or infiltrate the host's genetic apparatus, its deoxyribonucleic acid chains, to lie dormant until roused by some noxious stimulus. Though he had no way of knowing it at the time, the subject of virus-gene interactions has become a leading target of cancer researchers in the past two decades. The genital herpes virus—as opposed to the more benign type that causes fever sores on the lip when ac-

tivated by ultraviolent radiation from the sun—is now a prime
suspect as a causative agent in male and female genital carcinoma.)

Good received his M.D. and his Ph.D. in 1947, interning at the
university's hospital and taking his specialist residency there in
pediatrics. He chose the field because defects in the lymph-gland
immunologic defense system almost invariably make their
presence known in the young, the patients rarely surviving to
maturity because of the infections—and occasionally tumors—
that overwhelm them. Good has said, besides, "I like kids.
They're tough."

The young pediatrician, anatomist, microbiologist, and pathologist had progressed to American Legion Memorial research
professor of Pediatrics at Minnesota by 1954, having spent his
only time away from Minneapolis as a visiting investigator at
the Rockefeller University in the academic year 1949–50. He
was putting his name to a prodigious number of research reports
each year, and by the time the 1960s transplants came along
Good was in the forefront of investigation in that challenging
area. His credo was and continues to be "Learn from the patient
all he has to teach." His interest in the thymus gland stemmed
in part from his treatment of a patient whose continuing bouts
of infection seemed to be in some way related to a tumor of
the small gland.

Good received the Albert Lasker Medical Research award in
1970 for his pioneering work in understanding how the white
blood cell system of lymph-gland surveillance was armed and
cocked with the aid of the thymus gland, a mysterious little knot
of cells near the juncture of the neck and the chest, and also for
his clinical daring in the transplantation of bone marrow where
all the vital formed components of the blood are made, red cells
to carry oxygen and platelets for clotting as well as the defensive
white cells. Marrow grafts can be lifesaving for babies born
without the ability to produce white cells that manufacture antibodies. The disease is called congenital agammaglobulinemia
because immunologists generally refer to antibodies as immune
globulins. Good figured that marrow grafting, in which the
physician wipes out the young patient's ability to make all blood

components and then injects marrow from—usually—a near rela-
tive would be an exception to the rule that immune-suppressing
drugs or serums must be used to keep the patient from rejecting
the graft, as commonly practiced in kidney transplants. After
all, the graft here *was* the core of the rejecting system,
and a "take" would really reconstitute not only the infant's cell
type but his or her total concept, biologically, of what was self
and what was non-self. Marrow grafting, immunologically speak-
ing, produces a chimera when it is successful, a child who is
partly himself as he was born, but in an important respect
partly somebody else. Good was more concerned with "rejection"
of the patient by the graft. (This reaction is now known as
GVH for "graft-versus-host.") In 1966 he performed a reconsti-
tution, transplanting a billion marrow cells from a sister's thigh
bone into the belly of five-month-old David Camp who, lacking
a normal immune system, was unable to defend himself against
bacteria, viruses, and fungi. This made possible the boy's survival
even though the graft was not from an identical twin. (The
sister, one of four, was the best match, however.) David now
carries in his blood white cells characteristic of his sister. Since
mature platelets and red cells do not replicate and therefore do
not have chromosomes, only David's white cells bear the telltale
double X female chromosomes pair showing he is a chimera.
Good stuck by his guns after the intraperitioneal injection of
bone marrow cells homed into the infant's marrow, settled
there, grew, and produced a classic GVH syndrome. Relying on
mouse experiments he had performed a decade before, Good
refused to panic. Eventually the GVH reaction subsided and
David's sister's immune cells decided in some mysterious way
that they could accommodate their new host even though they
knew, again in some form of biological recognition not well
understood, that he was not their proper owner. Now they perform the normal defensive role of the immune system. Good,
these days, mentions David Camp in many contexts, the healthy
child that he most certainly saved from certain immunologically
deficient death.

Good has continued his quest for the genetic secrets that will
make such infant transplants more feasible. Not every child born

with an immunodeficiency disease like David Camp's has a well-matched sibling, or, indeed, any brother or sister at all. The progress made in identifying tissue incompatibilities now leads Good to predict that out of a pool of tissue-typed volunteers (comparable to the pools of rare blood-type volunteers needed for certain transfusions) he will be able to recruit marrow donors for the doomed infants. Such clinical research has enormous implications for cancer therapy. Since patients whose immune systems fail to work properly are ten times more likely to develop cancer than people whose immune systems are intact, scientists believe that a normal immune response acts as a barrier to cancer. If correction of immunodeficiency in patients could reduce their cancer toll, this would bolster the contention that a contributory cause of cancer is defective immunity. Marrow transplants are today being employed with some success in leukemia patients where drugs have ultimately failed to control the white-cell cancer.

In 1969 Good achieved his major goal at Minnesota, the Regents professorship of pediatrics and microbiology. He has said, "A proper administrator achieves with really successful administration the creation of a research professorship for himself. I'd really been able to administer my department so that now I could function not as an administrator but as a scholar and scientist."

In the midst of these achievements of the 1960s, Good was divorced by his wife and the mother of his five children. In 1967 he married a scientist who was, perhaps, better equipped to understand the long lab and office hours he keeps. Joanne Finstad Good, a geneticist interested in the evolution of traits and capabilities, now shares the Sloan-Kettering director's penthouse and, according to Good, can take much of the credit for getting him there. Not that Joanne Good isn't capable of engineering a coup or two of her own. Her husband credits her with supervising his and his associates' move from Minneapolis to New York. But in the case of Good's elevation to the top rank of New York's East Side medical establishment, Joanne played a very direct and vigorous role.

In the winter of 1971–72, Memorial Hospital's board chairman

Benno Schmidt had coaxed Good into becoming one of the triumvirate of former President Richard M. Nixon's special panel of advisers on the nation's new cancer program, along with Schmidt himself and Dr. R. Lee Clark, head of Houston's M. D. Anderson Hospital and Tumor Institute, a smaller but almost equally prestigious cancer center compared with Memorial Sloan-Kettering. The Memorial trustees, in particular Harold ("Bud") Fisher, one of Standard Oil's (Exxon's) two traditional members of the Center's board of trustees and then chairman of the Sloan-Kettering board, Laurance Rockefeller, chairman of the center, and Schmidt had asked Dr. Frank Dixon, a noted immunologist at the Scripps Clinic and Research Foundation in La Jolla, California, to become the Sloan-Kettering director. Good knew of this offer through Dixon and thus knew that the New Yorkers were looking for an immunologist.

Good had come to Memorial as guest lecturer a few months before, in 1971, and had probably sensed that he was to be tapped after Dixon. When Dixon turned the job down, the wooing of Good began. The public is not generally aware that scientists, like the rest of us, are fond of a little Puligny-Montrachet and nicely poached salmon, rounded off with a twenty-year-old cognac on occasion. One may be certain that Robert and Joanne Good's reception in New York City in late 1971 and early 1972 was different from that which the Rockefeller Institute visiting investigator had received a score of years before.

By March of 1972 the offer had been made and the time for decision was at hand. The Goods left Minneapolis for their vacation in Florida. Behind them was the farm in Monticello, forty miles out of town, their constant and beloved retreat from the pressures of Good's dual university posts and from the constant pressures and requests for seminars, speeches, and travel. Back there, too, were Good's second and third sons and his youngest child, a daughter, then a sophomore in high school. But Robert Good felt challenged by the kind of patients he would see at the New York cancer center—leukemias that might be candidates for marrow transplant and other more bizarre malignancies which he rarely encountered in Minneapolis. Joanne Good was evidently ready for the big city as well.

Nevertheless, Good told Joanne with an audible sigh a few days before St. Patrick's Day, he had decided to stay with his roots. His wife did not return to Minneapolis on the same flight with her husband. Having said "no" to Rockefeller on St. Patrick's Day, Good shortly said "maybe" and then said he would like a professorship at the board chairman's family university. That arranged, he said "yes."

By the time Good had installed Summerlin as the youngest full member of the Sloan-Kettering Institute, the six-foot-one South Carolinian had made a name for himself in the field of transplantation. There were some doubters though. A senior scientist at the New York Blood Center, a block from the Memorial Sloan-Kettering complex of buildings, was asked about Summerlin's arrival on the New York scene.

"Yes," said the scientist in his strong Slavic accent, "I remember he came over here to our immunology laboratories. Your Dr. Summerlin was a very charming and persuasive man. When he left, I said, 'No, we do not want to work with that man.' And we did not."

Probably only an experienced scientist well endowed with intuition or else a very cynical and blasé layman would remain unconvinced if William Summerlin chose to make a believer of him. Like Good's brisk baritone, Summerlin's tenor drawl wrings enthusiasm from his listeners. Both men use a homely idiom with little jargon when they are talking to laymen. Both have the height to look anyone in the eye and rarely fail to do so. Neither could or would call any man Mr. or any woman Miss or Mrs. after the first three minutes of conversation. Their eyes offer a contrast, Good's hazel and heavy-lidded, deep set in his somewhat swarthy face, whereas Summerlin's brown irises, oddly, promise innocence and sincerity.

Good, a child of the depression, learned about finance companies and bill juggling early on. Summerlin's needs are those of the next generation raised amid financial security but often left emotionally adrift. Summerlin feeds on approbation, without it he starves. Good is more interested in the absolutes of success—the power and the perquisites, of course, but also the knowledge that he can change medical history.

Bill Summerlin was born to Lewis Findley and Joseph Talley Summerlin in Anderson, South Carolina, on December 6, 1938. Joseph Summerlin ran a dry cleaning business. His son worked at the YMCA off and on while attending the local public schools and received a scholarship to Emory University in Atlanta in 1955. He worked in the library as an undergraduate and married Rebecca the year before he graduated. At Emory's School of Medicine he was accused of cheating in an episode that made the local paper. Gail McBride, a news reporter for the *Journal of the American Medical Association,* learned in 1974 that the alleged cheating was in an examination during the extraordinarily tough sophmore year of medical school but that since Summerlin denied the charges and nothing could be proved, he was graduated with a clean slate.

Summerlin interned at the University of Texas Medical Branch in Galveston, then moved on to Fort Sam Houston and its famed Brooke Army Medical Center where surgical research is concentrated on burn therapy. The Army, of course, is extremely interested in learning how to counter the effects of phosphorus, flaming gasoline, napalm, and high explosives on the human epidermis, but Brooke also receives the scalded victims who are dependents of service men. In doing his residency at Brooke, Summerlin came in contact with a desperately sick group of patients for whom skin grafting—even on a temporary basis—can be lifesaving.

One doctor who worked with Summerlin during his sojourn with the Army center told Gail McBride, "Those of us who knew him felt he had made the best possible choice when he decided not to go into surgery." Said another, ". . . the burn and trauma unit was understaffed at the time, so that the maximum output was required of everyone. Dr. Summerlin didn't give that; he couldn't seem to adapt and adjust to what was required of him. Eventually he was transferred away from the burn patients to another part of the unit—to an environment with less pressure—and he seemed to do better there."

Once Summerlin had left Brooke and, in mid-1967, taken up a dermatology residency at Stanford University Medical Center, his career began to prosper. He had an NIH (National Institutes of Health) fellowship and his chief, Professor Eugene Farber, told Gail McBride, "Dr. Summerlin was an outstanding resident." In fact, Farber complained mildly to Bob Good when the latter accepted Summerlin's application to come to Minnesota four years later.

At Stanford, Summerlin encountered Marvin A. Karasek, Ph.D., who in 1966 had perfected a technique originally developed by a naval researcher for the growth in culture of fibroblasts and other living units of skin.

Karasek, queried by the author, wrote: "The work that Summerlin published with me while he was a student in my laboratory in 1968 was documented, appropriately supervised and has been reconfirmed both in our own laboratory and in others." The problem that obviously intrigued Summerlin at Stanford was whether the culture techniques that Karasek had developed could be clinically applied. Consider the victim of extensive burns who thereby requires extensive grafting to keep vital body fluids from leaking out of his or her exposed tissue and to keep bacteria from coming in. Summerlin must have wondered whether, perhaps, a small patch of skin might be encouraged to grow larger and thus provide multiple grafts that might seed hopelessly broad areas of scorched tissue with which the surgeon treating victims of explosions and scalding is often faced. In such instances doctors had in the past even resorted to pigskin, knowing full well that the porcine integument would be rapidly rejected but hoping to buy time for the patient's recovery from the devastating shock (lethal alterations in the sodium and potassium content of tissues and of blood flow) that can kill burn victims early, or at least to guard against the bacteria that can kill them later.

Summerlin was a physician; Karasek was not. Summerlin was therefore empowered by the state of California to slice judiciously a sector of skin from a volunteer's forearm or thigh, nourish it in a dish, and then carefully replace the living cells to see whether they had been compromised by their sojourn out of the body. It seemed they had not been, as Summerlin and Karasek reported to the *Journal of Investigative Dermatology* in March of 1970, a communication the journal published that November. As Summerlin later described this period in his research, "Beginning in 1967–68, a clinical study was begun which demonstrated that whole human skin maintained for extended periods of time in organ culture, though quite hypocellular [retaining few viable cells] at the time of transplant, did, indeed, function as normal fresh autograft when transplanted autologously after such periods of time in culture." The dermatologist was referring here to his removal and replacement of skin in the same individual. He went on, "It was thus realized that for the first time we had a model to study a whole viable organ [the skin] for extended periods in vitro in the laboratory."

But William Summerlin was neither by training nor inclination a man to set off down a painstaking path of animal research; that was obviously for the Ph.D.s like Karasek. Summerlin could see the potential of skin banks for ulcerated and severely burned human patients. Perhaps he could make a century-old fantasy come true by tissue culture. It was in Paris in 1867 that the Swiss surgeon Jacques Louis Reverdin became the first physician to practice the art of skin grafting. Reverdin found that if he cut under the outer, epidermal layer of living and dead cells and into the inner dermis, composed mainly of tough, interwoven collagen fibers, he could simply place the partly dermal and mostly epidermal section right on an open, unhealed wound, holding it in place with a tight bandage until continuity was reestablished between the patient's raw, wet tissue and the base of the graft.

Reverdin's report set off an orgy of grafting in which surgeons planted a variety of animal pelts onto human lesions in the expectation that they would grow and protect the patient. The bubble burst in 1911 when a German surgeon, Erich Lexer, demonstrated conclusively that these supposed skin grafts were, in fact, only dressings for wounds and that even the close relationship of parent and child could not overcome the propensity of the body to destroy alien transplanted skin.

In 1969 Summerlin set about the task of grafting skin on patients from unrelated donors, first growing the cells in culture for four to six weeks. Though Karasek does not choose to discuss the matter, it is apparent that the first of the series of personal frictions that were to mar the young skin specialist's sojourns in Palo Alto, Minneapolis, and New York erupted over the transplant matter. In the event, Summerlin took his project over to the Veterans Administration Hospital affiliated with Stanford, leaving his senior research collaborator behind and conspicuously omitting him from any authorship of the results he eventually published in the spring of 1973, having presented them at several meetings in the interim.

In attempting to breach a well-accepted medical dogma, most careful researchers would make every effort to protect themserves against any hint of prejudice. This is normally accomplished by what is called the "blind" technique of evaluation of results. The method is more widely used in new drug research than in surgery. The investigator presents to colleagues who are well equipped to assess them data on a series of patients, some of whom have been given the treatment under trial and others of whom have been treated by the older, established method upon which the researcher is trying to improve. The evaluating colleagues are not told which patients have received which treatment, so they can, presumably, be entirely objective in gauging the results. (In properly blind pharmaceutical testing, the researcher himself, in addition to the testers, is given pills or vials that are coded by number or color, the code being broken only after the patients' responses have been checked. This situation, in which neither doctor nor patient knows what is being given—new drug, older drug, or, perhaps, an inert sugar pill called a "placebo"—is termed "double-blind," but it is clearly not feasible where the surgeon must cut the patient.)

In Summerlin's clinical trial it would have been valuable to test the merits of cultivating donor A's skin before applying it to recipient B to make comparisions at the same site. One would have wanted to check A's cells cultured for a month against A's cells immediately transplanted and also against B's own cells from another part of B's body, which would have been expected to succeed. Thus if B's cells failed to establish themselves at the graft site, the technique of transplant and not the rejection phenomenon would be to blame. If, on the other hand, the freshly taken cells from A failed to thrive while the cultured cells from A and the freshly taken cells from B did well, this would constitute strong evidence for the hypothesis Summerlin was advancing, that organs could be successfully transplanted between genetically incompatible people. Finally, of course, the dermatologist could have added one more safeguard by adding to the permutations B's own cells that had been grown in culture. In treating his first four patients, Summerlin reported, he chose a three-graft plan, cultured and fresh skin from an unmatched donor (or cadaver) and a fresh, uncultured graft from some other area of the patient's body, each about the size of a postage stamp.

Though in this first report he makes it clear that he deliberately exchanged skin cells between sexes so that the Barr body (the sex chromatin) might serve as a marker, and though he says the chromosomal analysis was conducted independently by a colleague, Summerlin does not specify the stain that was used. In any case, he served as operator, judge, and jury in determining which of the three patches of skin survived and which were rejected. He also judged that the epidermis of the four patients showed no signs of regenerative capability, that there was no growth from the edges of the wound or lesion toward its center, indicating absence of a spontaneous healing process before the grafting.

Summerlin reported that the freshly cut and grafted tissue from a stranger was rejected after about two weeks. But, he said, the cultured cells stayed on, along with the cells taken from another part of the patient's own body. He did not wait until his data had been published to report this stunning news, and word of the skin transplant successes spread rapidly in medical circles around the nation.

Summerlin and Good met at a dermatology research meeting in Miami in December of 1969 where Good, an indefatigable guest speaker, had given a lecture. Summerlin made the approach. He said later, "I introduced myself and said I was interested in immunology. We had breakfast the next morning and

he invited me to Minnesota, but I said it was probably premature." Within eighteen months, however, Summerlin had decided
the time was ripe and contacted Good, the proprietor of one of
the nation's largest immunologic research groups, one that was
itself virtually a satellite medical center.

The move would be to the advantage of both parties. Good
had money to support Summerlin's research and Summerlin apparently had a major transplantation breakthrough but no
research support of his own. The first Summerlin paper to which
Good added his name, for example, lists support for the animal
experimentation from the National Institutes of Health, the U. S.
Public Health Service, the Veterans Administration, and the National Foundation (March of Dimes).

When Summerlin applied to Good, though, the senior scientist, who had struggled for years for every nickel of grant and
salary money he got, found the applicant's optimistic improvi-
dence distressing. Dr. Summerlin had no grant of his own? Summerlin wasn't worried about that. He wanted to work with Good.
Good agreed to take the dermatologist, but he silently bridled
at this carefree attitude.

Summerlin left Palo Alto for Minneapolis in August 1971. Good
allotted him a technician and laboratory space in his quarters
atop the Variety Club Heart Hospital and sent the young doctor
around to visit with more experienced transplantation investigators in the Minnesota group so that Summerlin could learn the
various techniques and disciplines of animal transplantation in
what was surely one of the nation's most sophisticated centers for
such experimentation. After that, Summerlin worked mostly
alone, using his own mouse colony and not drawing upon the
highly pedigreed animals from the Minneapolis medical school's
central colonies in another building. This combination of solo
work and the use of mice not formally certified by the physiology
department as to pedigree was to loom large in the later investigation of Summerlin's claimed successes.

3

bAptism ANd TEMptATioN

BY THE END of March in 1973 Summerlin had found
the Darien house for his family and was beginning to cope with
his new milieu at the New York cancer center. But on March 29
he left his hectic schedule behind to board an American Airlines
jet bound for Tucson, Arizona. After two winters in the cold
climate of Minneapolis and New York, the Southerner was looking forward to the warmth of Arizona. Though the trip was for
business, very important business with the American Cancer So-

ciety, Bill Summerlin was anticipating some relaxed hours in the
sunshine of the Southwest.

But instead of the expected mellow temperature after the six-
hour flight, he found that the mercury in Arizona had collapsed
into the forties, the skies were leaden, and snowflakes appeared
from time to time as he drove with a newly made acquaintance
to a motel just north of Nogales and the Mexican border. Jerry
Bishop, a veteran science reporter for *The Wall Street Journal,*
had taken the same jet from New York and was glad to accommodate a fellow traveler in his rented car. But after a brief conversation about the unexpected weather, the dialogue lapsed and
Bishop was unable to revive it. Later, William Summerlin would
prove affable, even loquacious, with the press, but with Bishop
he restrained his habitual camaraderie. The reporter was later to
wonder whether his passenger had mistaken him for a colleague
in research and hence to be treated with some discretion. Bishop
knew, however, that Summerlin was a protégé of Good. He knew
also that the physician was shortly to appear with a couple of
dozen cancer researchers in a six-day marathon of presentations
to the medical and science writers of the nation's leading mold-
ers of opinion, its news magazines, wire services, newspapers, and
radio and television networks.

The assembly at the new Rio Rico Inn in Nogales, was the
fifteenth such annual conclave for science writers sponsored by
the American Cancer Society, on whose scientific board Robert
Good occupied a prominent place. If Good said Summerlin was
ready for the Arizona sunshine of publicity, then he was. In addition, Summerlin had reason to hope that his presentation and
resulting articles about it in the public press and on radio and
television might influence favorably a grant application he had
made earlier in the month to the society requesting support for
his research. If he got the full amount sought, his laboratory at
Sloan-Kettering would receive $131,564 over a five-year period.

Both the timing and the location of the Nogales meeting had
been carefully chosen by Alan Davis, then newly named to a
vice-presidency in the cancer society. Davis, whose boyishly
handsome features and jocular attitude when in the presence of
reporters conceal a meticulous attention to protocol and detail,

knew that the news of progress against cancer coming out of
Arizona should break coincident with the start of the society's
fund-raising month on April 1. He also knew that by decree of
his predecessor and inventor of the reporters' cancer seminar, a
keg of a man named Patrick McGrady, the locale should be a
warm and sunny one calculated to lure writers from New York
and Chicago and Minneapolis and Kansas City where winter's
lease often extends to Easter. The westerlies had played Davis
false, but then even a vice-president encounters factors beyond
his control.

McGrady, a native of Montana who had worked for Bernarr
Macfadden's New York *Evening Graphic* and covered news of
China out of Shanghai in the 1940s, proposed to the cancer society in 1947 that a reportorial tour of selected laboratories funded
by it would create in the American people an impression of bus-
tling activity and forward movement against the disease that
would impel the public hand toward its pocket. The next spring,
eight carefully selected writers from the three wire services, and
such dailies as the New York *Times* and New York *Herald
Tribune,* the Washington *Post,* and the Chicago *Tribune* set off
on the ten-day tour, taking notes on ten to twelve presentations
in a city in the morning and writing their articles in the afternoon before leaving for the next stop. In those days, when newspaper competition within major cities pitted morning paper reporters against their afternoon rivals with unbridled ferocity, it
was deemed necessary by McGrady to keep the peace on the
road by the technique known as a news embargo. In other
words, the first six reports given were arbitrarily allotted to the
morning newspaper reporters and to the wire service writers for
Associated Press, United Press, and International News Service
on a schedule that would be available for their morning paper
subscribers. The next five or six reports, even though capable of
being reported for morning papers, were reserved for the afternoon papers. That practice is still honored today, though the
tour, grown to more than fifty reporters, succumbed to logistical
hysteria in 1959. "Guys were coming and going," McGrady has
said, "and we just couldn't keep track of the transportation and
hotel room permutations. So we decided to put the whole thing

under one roof, and we figured in the cold wind of March, who
could resist Phoenix or La Jolla or St. Augustine?" Few major
news media did, even though, as on presidential and other political campaign junkets, room and transport bills were and are paid
by the media. (This rule is violated only for a handful of
selected small-town newspapers, changed each year, whose reporters are invited to attend "on the house.")

Over the twenty-six years of its existence, the cancer tour has
served both the society and the reporters well, assuring the
former of valuable headlines helpful to fund raising and the latter access to leading researchers both formally during the tightly
scheduled sessions and informally at the ninety-minute "happy
hour" starting at five-thirty, when Messrs. McGrady and Davis
provide 86-proof lubrication for minds made sluggish by ac-
cumulated research data.

There are some in both the scientific and journalistic fraterni-
ties, however, who question the neatly packaged procedure.
What is missing, they aver, is the vigorous questioning that
follows any scientific report that breaks new ground or calls into
question an accepted tenet. Because the programs of national
and local medical and scientific society meetings are published in
advance, there is a virtual guarantee that the audience for a particular report will contain many scientists and doctors who specialize in that field. Thus the questioning of the reporting scientist will be both sharp and sophisticated and may well bring to
light flaws in the experiment or in the conclusions drawn from it
by the investigator. Such flaws are not easily spotted by science
and medicine reporters, who normally have to cover all of medicine, psychology, astrophysics, etc.

For example, a decade ago, a psychologist interested in the
biochemical mechanism of learning described an experiment in
which, apparently, a flatworm called a planarian appeared to
learn faster as a result of being fed bits of other planaria that
had undergone a simple training program. The psychologist's colleagues in that area jumped out of their seats as soon as he had
finished. They suggested half a dozen ways in which the experiment was flawed and in which other conclusions could have been
reached.

By the nature of the cancer writers' seminars this sort of prob-
ing is, at best, considerably diluted. Cancer research covers a
wide range of scientific disciplines, so that even if all of the invited researchers were present to hear each presentation with the
reporters—which they are not—there would be few qualified to
question in detail the procedures and conclusions presented. In
addition, since all are invited guests of the American Cancer Society, there would be a natural reluctance to come down hard on
a fellow guest's report that had been precertified by Davis and
the society's research board.

In such situations, conscientious reporters faced with novel or
controversial data normally seek out their own trusted consultants in the reported field either by prowling the corridors or by
using long-distance telephone. This solution to the checking
problem is normally feasible at annual cancer seminars, but in
the case of Summerlin's report of successful transplantation without resorting to drugs or sera to suppress rejection, this avenue
was, by chance, effectively shut off.

McGrady had recognized two immutable facts of press
agentry: never break a big story on Friday because the circulation of most daily newspapers is drastically reduced on Saturday;
and break your best stories early on Saturday because Sunday
morning newspapers achieve peak circulation figures and there
are no Sunday afternoon papers. However, since McGrady had
also known that weekends are news poor and that editors could
best spare their reporters on Friday, Saturday, and Sunday, he
had had to include these days in his six-day week. His solution
had been to start the presentations on Friday afternoon with
generalizations from the officialdom of the government and the
society that could either be written for the meager Saturday
circulation or held for feature use at the end of the seminar.
Thus were supposed losers devoid of hard, "breakthrough" news
quarantined for the Saturday few.

At the Nogales meeting in 1973, Davis compromised this tactic
to a degree, starting his batting order at 3:00 P.M. on Friday,
March 30, with a welcome by the Arizona Secretary of State and
a president's report by Dr. Arthur G. James of the Ohio State
University School of Medicine, head of the cancer society.

Next on the program, however, was Summerlin's presentation, titled without any apparent reservations "Organ Transplant Without Immunosupression." It came at 3:20 P.M., Texas time. Reporters at the meeting, a vast majority of whom had covered the disspiriting results of heart transplants in the years immediately preceding the Nogales meeting, were told that a potential way around graft rejection had been found. Said Summerlin: ". . . I found that after human skin is maintained in organ culture for four to six weeks, it becomes universally transplantable without rejection." Not content with this remarkably unreserved assertion, Summerlin went on to promise other bonuses: "We have since attempted to extend this work to other organ systems and find that whole cornea from a number of species, human included, functions quite normally during the culture process and is transplantable without rejection (xenogeneically and allogeneically) into rabbit-eye recipients. Moreover, work with other organs, including the mouse adrenal gland, shows that such organs maintain their function during organ culture and after critical periods of time in vitro (in glassware), take allogeneically without rejection and function quite normally after such transplantation . . ."

This was a tasty dish for a Friday afternoon, and, since it had been designated for Saturday morning newspapers, there was little or no time for any reporter for newspapers east of the Rocky Mountains to digest it. Summerlin was saying that growing skin and other cells in laboratory glassware and in special nutrients for a brief period somehow cancelled the effects of their identifying chemical markers (antigens) that would cause rejection if they were taken directly from one animal and transplanted into another. Furthermore, he was saying that this was true not only allogeneically (within species of different genetic stock) but also "xenogeneically (across the lines of orders, or "from man to mouse," in the common phraseology).

After four to six weeks in culture, he related, as he had before his peers at the meeting of the Transplantation Society in San Francisco the previous September, skin cells from unrelated donors had survived as grafts on four patients for more than a year.

The science writers, faced with a transplantation "break-through" of major proportions, had to make a choice in a hurry. On the one hand, a good news story on the first day of the meeting would demonstrate to their editors back home that they were earnestly in search of news and not just taking life easy. In addition, writing this story would be easier than some complicated piece of hamster or guinea pig research without immediate application to human patients. Summerlin, after all, had *started* with human patients, so the application was apparent. Also, every reporter for a tight-budget paper was aware that if he sent a readily comprehensible article on the first day of the meeting, he or she would be in a stronger position on the next day to send along a more complex research story.

Against the Summerlin findings was the obvious fact that they had little to do with cancer research, though the Sloan-Kettering doctor made his obeisances to his hosts: "These observations do offer a model for host-tumor relationships and provide a significant link between transplantation and cancer immunology."

The strongest assets for the story were the well-known facts that Good, a personal favorite of most writers at Nogales for his ready accessibility, was backing Summerlin and had brought him from Minneapolis to Sloan-Kettering.

This was not enough for the Associated Press and United Press International reporters, who, lacking any way to put the magic word "cancer" in their first sentences, chose silence. It was, however, plenty for such experienced hands as Philip Brimble of the Kansas City *Star* (SKIN GRAFT TRANSPLANT GAIN) and Arthur Page of the Buffalo *Evening News* (SKIN BANKS SOME DAY MAY AID BURN VICTIMS). A news story on Summerlin's achievement was also syndicated by the Hearst Headline Service to the Hearst chain of dailies.

But the most important personage weighing the Summerlin account was a small, intense young woman, amply endowed with the experience and knowledge to sniff out a green or overripe report, given to contentious questions, and well aware that her newspaper, the New York *Times,* never forgot or forgave an embarrassment. It had been arranged that Jane Brody and a medical reporter for the Baltimore *News American,* Joanne Rodgers,

would have lunch with Summerlin before he made his presentation. Both had in hand the three-page summary of the report he
would give that afternoon. Both reporters were used to writing
news stories about Good's rare but successful bone marrow transplants and his many other notable achievements in medical science. They had also brought to the Rio Rico lunch table the
knowledge that Good had only recently stepped down as one of
President Nixon's trio of top advisers on implementation of the
country's newly declared all-out war against cancer. Dr. Summerlin might as well have had stamped on his high, sallow forehead
some such inscription as "Merchandise certified and guaranteed
by Robert A. Good, M.D., Ph.D.," as far as the ladies at his
lunch table were concerned.

Jane Brody later recalled Summerlin's charm and enthusiasm
as he vividly told them that the cultures of human skin cells "had
looked like hell" before they were placed on his patients' unhealing ulcers. She said, "He wasn't exactly my type but he was very,
very persuasive."

By the time the young dermatologist rose to talk to the assembled science reporters, typesetters at the *Times* were already
casting the lead for the story that ran the next day under a three-
column headline on page 50. Partly because of the two-hour time
differential between Arizona and New York, partly because of
Good's high regard for Summerlin and his seeming breach of
the immunologic barrier that had decimated the ranks of heart
transplant patients, Jane Brody did not contact other leaders in
the field of organ grafting. Under the headline LAB DISCOVERY
MAY AID TRANSPLANTS, readers of Saturday's *Times* would find
no hint in the story about Summerlin's work and its significance
of the caveats that normally mark Brody's treatment of new medical developments and, indeed, those of most wary reporters.

Although the *Times* editors played the story far back in the
newspaper, Summerlin was now clearly launched as a scientific
celebrity, albeit of the second rank. As one moneygatherer at
Memorial Sloan-Kettering later put it, "We all knew he was a hot
property."

Once that three-column headline appeared in the *Times,* medical editors for *Time* and *Newsweek* and many another national

magazine could be certain of a visit or a memo from a higher rung on the editorial ladder, inquiring, "Are we looking into this breakthrough in transplantation I read about in the *Times* last Saturday?" *Newsweek's* medical editor was at the Nogales meeting and kept the ball rolling with a story and a picture of a Summerlin black mouse wearing a white skin patch under the headline "New Help for Skin Grafts," on April 23. *Saturday Review/World* blurted "Cultured Organs" in its next science issue.

Summerlin, meanwhile, was off on a round of medical meetings to which he would bring his immunologic tidings. At the May meeting in Atlantic City of the American Society for Clinical Investigation, a notably fussy group that, in medical circles, bears the long-outdated nickname "Young Turks," Summerlin embroidered some further stitching, duly reported by the publication *Medical Tribune* the following month. He now spoke of experiments involving the pancreas, the thymus gland, and other unspecified organs served by large blood vessels, and he continued to assert that mice did not reject adrenal glands for at least six months if the glands were nourished outside the animals' bodies beforehand. As for grafts of corneas, Summerlin said human tissue grown in culture had been accepted by rabbits and had endured for six months, whereas corneas freshly cut out and immediately transplanted from cadavers to rabbits were rejected by the recipient animals in six weeks. The coauthors listed for this paper were Dr. Good and Dr. George E. Miller, a research fellow and resident in ophthalmology at the University of Minnesota Hospitals.

Miller's and Good's names had already appeared on an earlier Summerlin report on the feasibility of culturing—as opposed to simply refrigerating—corneas in the March issue of the journal *Investigative Ophthalmology*. But in addition to their names and that of Dr. Summerlin, there appeared that of Dr. John E. Harris, professor and head of the University of Minnesota Department of Ophthalmology.

Harris later asserted without qualification that no corneal experiments undertaken by him or by his resident, Miller, could in any way justify Summerlin's conclusions proclaimed to the Young Turks that the eye tissue grafted more effectively after culture in vitro for several weeks.

As the head of a laboratory at the Sloan-Kettering Institute, Summerlin was, in the summer of 1973, amassing a considerable staff. He had four secretaries to aid him in running the hospital's skin clinic, in making his applications for grants, in typing his reports, and in administering research that employed half a dozen postdoctoral research fellows—surgeons, dermatologists, and immunologists who wanted to train under Good and who chose to work for Summerlin because of his reports of extraordinary progress in an area that had been exasperating the best medical brains in the world.

In addition to these considerable resources, Summerlin was able to call upon talent at the Cornell University Medical College-New York Hospital complex. Since Sloan-Kettering is affiliated with Cornell (many of the members and associate members hold faculty posts with the university), it was easily arranged that two New York Hospital-Cornell ophthalmologists should take up the corneal transplant work where it had been dropped when Summerlin left Minnesota. The Cornell eye specialists had, however, not yet begun their experiments with Sloan-Kettering rabbits when Summerlin was expatiating on his corneal graft successes in Atlantic City.

In its slow, methodical fashion, the world of medical science had begun to respond to Summerlin's speeches and publications in the second half of 1973. Laboratories from Amsterdam to London and from North Carolina to Colorado were systematically slicing skin from hordes of mice, soaking the harvest in special media often enriched with calf's blood and antibiotics, letting the soup incubate, and then troweling it onto meticulously wounded animals of genetically incompatible strains. The results were uniform and dreary. Black mice rejected skin from white mice. Agoutis sloughed gray skin. Albino animals destroyed black epidermis. As fall chilled to gray November, a parade of junior researchers from Duke University, the University of Colorado, the Shriners' Burns Institute in Boston, and the Radiobiological Institute in The Netherlands arrived on Sixty-eighth Street, seeking from Summerlin some hint as to technique, some unmentioned ingredient in the nutrient medium, some post-operative dressing that could account for his success and their failures. The visitors were uniformly spun off by Summerlin to the postdoctoral fellows. Letters from their home labs went unanswered. Summerlin was furiously busy with patients, administrative details, and, most of all, with his applications for support.

The arrival of Good at Sloan-Kettering had been widely accepted as a sharp turn for the Memorial Sloan-Kettering Cancer Center, a corporate entity formed in 1968 to co-ordinate bookkeeping, fund raising, and administration for the institute and hospital. He had brought with him from the Minnesota campus fifty men and women with degrees and advanced capabilities in the relatively new specialty of immunology. Now was the time for the ultraconservative Sloan-Kettering Institute, which had been founded in 1945, to take a fresh direction, expand its research efforts in consonance with the nation's expanded campaign to control cancer, and, highest priority of all, to raise the funds that would support a 75 per cent increase in the research budget. If this mandate was made clear to Good, it was made equally clear to subordinate researchers that they were to get cracking on the grants and compete actively for the largesse flowing, albeit sporadically, for the pseudo-Georgian campus of the National Institutes of Health in Bethesda, Maryland, and, more specifically, from the National Cancer Institute of the NIH with its then $500-million annual federal grant for cancer research.

While Summerlin could and did shrug off the visits of the puzzled researchers who had tried and failed to duplicate his transplantation successes, there was one scientist who was not so easily put off. Sir Peter Medawar was a member of the board of scientific consultants of Sloan-Kettering, a group of about twenty distinguished researchers from leading institutions around the world who gather at the institute periodically to review its programs and projects and to offer their suggestions and criticisms about work in progress.

Dr. Medawar had been working for many years, first at University College in London and subsequently as director of Britain's justly famed National Institute for Medical Research, on precisely the problem with which the Summerlin project was concerned. In 1960 he had been awarded a Nobel prize in medicine for his work on the problem of graft-rejection mechanisms and some complex means by which the process could be prevented. (In the 1950s Dr. Medawar and Dr. Rupert Billingham, now at the Southwestern Medical School in Dallas, Texas, and Leslie Brent, now professor of zoology at the University of London, had shown that if one injected a newborn mouse with cells from an animal of a different strain, one could, later in life, apply a graft to the injected mouse from the cell-donor mouse and it would take. The process is called "induction of tolerance," but of course, it has no immediate application to human medicine. It simply proved that certain immune mechanisms can be influenced when they are not yet fully developed as they are in the mature mouse and in all mature vertebrates except for certain very primitive fishes.)

Medawar, hearing of Summerlin's success, had set some of his juniors to repeating the procedure, and, like the other investigators from other medical centers, had been given only negative reports. He made known his doubts at a meeting of the Sloan-Kettering consultants on October 14, 1973.

The scientific advisers, including such renowned immunologists as Dr. Dixon of Scripps and Rockefeller University's Dr. Henry Kunkel, had been listening to a number of presentations on projects by various Sloan-Kettering researchers. This was a session intended partly to replace the usual review by peers, to which, thanks to the lump-sum annual National Cancer Institute grants of funds to Sloan-Kettering Institute, Sloan-Kettering scientists rarely had to submit. It had been an exciting afternoon, according to Good, and then it was Summerlin's turn.

"There was a lot of clanking in the hall outside," Good recalled, "and whole cages were moved in. I had asked Summerlin to make a presentation at that meeting. He brought the mice with the handsome white grafts on them, the brown mice, and then at the end the rabbits with the corneal transplants from human cadavers, and after he had made the presentation, I said, 'And those are limbus-to-limbus [complete, edge-to-edge] corneal transplants,' and I made it clear that this was a fantastic thing.

Because when you transplant corneas limbus to limbus, the site isn't priviledged, isn't protected from destruction by white cells in the blood as it would be if you put a piece of cornea in the middle of the eye where it isn't adjacent to any blood supply. I still have nightmares about those remarks of mine. And then Dr. Prunieras got up and he presented his mice from Paris. [Dr. Michel Prunieras of the Rothschild Foundation in Paris had just written a letter to *Science* in which he had reported that, though he couldn't see prolonged mouse skin graft takes when he used the transplantation technique of Medawar, Brent, and Billingham, he was achieving sixty to seventy-five-day takes when he adjusted the procedure according to Summerlin's instructions. The letter was published by *Science* on November 2.] These mice confirmed the Summerlin observations, but that was the first I had seen of those mice. Prunieras is a very responsible scientist and a member of the French National Academy, and I had brought him here to check Summerlin's work. He presented some black mice with some nice tufts of white hair on them. Our method at Minnesota that I had asked one of our scientists to teach Summerlin was an adaptation of the Medawar-Brent-Billingham method and this was the first I'd heard of Summerlin using a different technique, that of the 'physiological dressing.' At Minnesota our people would go down through the dermis [skin] to the muscle and scarify it to make a really vascular graft bed [with a rich blood supply] and then lay in the graft. Summerlin was covering this graft with skin taken from a mouse of the same strain as the recipient, a syngeneic graft. Anyway, even with Prunieras' report, Dr. Medawar was still very skeptical. 'Tufts of white hair,' he said. 'You can get tufts of white hair in all sorts of ways.' Anybody that's done transplantation knows the hazard of white on black because of loss of the melanin pigmentation during healing. But I thought the session ended with Dixon and Kunkel and Medawar quite convinced that Summerlin had a real phenomenon in hand."

The rabbits Summerlin exhibited that day, he said, had undergone corneal transplants by Drs. Peter Laino and Bartley Mondino, the two Cornell-New York Hospital ophthalmologists. One member of Summerlin's audience at the scientific advisers' meet-

ing was especially interested in his description of the rabbits.
Summerlin averred that one eye of each rabbit had been grafted
with corneal tissue freshly removed from a human cadaver,
while the other eye had been grafted with cornea from the same
corpse but one that had been grown in culture for several weeks.
In both animals exhibited, one eye was functioning normally
while the other was opacified by rejection of the transplant. Summerlin claimed that the good eyes were those into which the cultured tissue had been stitched.

The intrigued observer was a young, sandy-haired postdoctoral
fellow from Summerlin's group who had given up a teaching career at the University of Utah to join Good's institution. With
a Ph.D. in immunology from Colorado State University, Dr. John
L. Ninnemann had naturally chosen to correspond with Dr. Summerlin about a post at Sloan-Kettering and he had joined the
staff on the customary date for fellows to assume their posts, July
1, that year.

The bespectacled young scientist had come to New York not
intending to learn if genetically incompatible transplants could
be made to work after tissue culture but why it worked. However, communications from other laboratories had been worrying
Good—though not muting his enthusiastic endorsement of Summerlin's results—and so, during the summer of 1973, Ninnemann,
with the help of Summerlin's transplantation technician, had set
about denuding and reconstituting a large collection of black,
white, gray, and speckled mice with pieces of each other's pelts.

During this process, he frequently had occasion to take the
mice into a surgical chamber on the eleventh floor of the Kettering Laboratory. From the animal quarters next door, Ninnemann
would carry the carefully tagged shiny, metal bins containing the
rodents, to change their dressings or take tiny samples of the
grafted tissue growing on their flanks.

Ninnemann later recalled: "Sometimes the New York-Cor-
nell ophthalmologists were in there at the same time and we'd
talk, naturally, about the work we were doing. It was in one of
those sessions that I learned from Dr. Bartley Mondino that they
were culturing corneal cells and then grafting one eye of each
rabbit.

"It would seem that the best way to compare rejection of a fresh cornea with rejection of cultured corneas would be to insert one in one eye and one in the other. But aside from humane reasons of possibly blinding the animal, there is a good immunologic reason for having separate control animals and operating on only one eye. When you put fresh incompatible cornea into one eye, you would sensitize the animal to such an extent that it would be virtually certain to reject your cultured cornea when it was placed in the other eye. So they had two groups of rabbits, one to receive fresh, the other cultured corneas in only one eye.

"So they started the work with the fresh corneas in September. By the time the Sloan-Kettering board of scientific advisers met in October, they still had not done the cultured corneas. Dr. Summerlin was called upon to report on his work at the advisers' conference. I had some mouse skin grafts that were evidently surviving eighteen days after transplantation and Dr. Summerlin wanted me to bring those over to show the board. He had an old mouse from Minnesota and some rats that were passed around and two rabbits, which he proceeded to describe as having gotten two grafts, fresh cornea on one side and cultured cornea on the other. Sir Peter Medawar was there and expressed the objection that this was nothing very extraordinary since the cornea isn't laced with blood vessels and thus has no supply of white blood cells of the type that destroy incompatible grafts. Dr. Good assured Dr. Medawar that the way the experiment was being conducted, the grafts were put into the rabbits' eyes from limbus to limbus and were, therefore, exposed to blood circulation."

(The limbus is simply a scientific term for the periphery or edge of the eye, and the reader has only to stand in front of a mirror and pull his or her lid away from the cornea to verify that the periphery of the eye is rendered scarlet by the presence of tiny arteries and veins. The redness seen in the eye after straining, sleeplessness, sleep, excessive drinking, or smoking marijuana comes from the dilation of vessels well beneath the cornea, those that serve the retinal cells within the eye.)

Good was mistaken in what he told Medawar, however. Mondino says that the rabbit transplants were not limbus to limbus. The immune reaction when order lines are crossed, as in these man-to-rabbit grafts, is so strong that blood vessels grow gradually into the cornea enabling destructive white cells eventually to get at the transplant and destroy it.

Ninnemann continued: "The statement by Dr. Summerlin about the clear eye and the cloudy eye disturbed me because I had talked to Dr. Mondino a week or so earlier and recalled his saying that only one eye had been grafted. So I called Dr. Mondino on the phone [after the science advisers' meeting] and he confirmed the one-side graft. So here was Dr. Summerlin showing a rabbit's eye that hadn't been grafted at all and saying it was an example of how cultured cornea wouldn't be rejected like fresh cornea. So I confronted Dr. Summerlin on this and he said 'No, no, I'm sure you're mistaken. I know they were grafted on both sides. Let's go up to the animal room and I'll show you.' So we went through every cage there and we could not find any animal in which both sides had been grafted, because you would see suture lines either way.

"After going through this, he said, 'Well, maybe I'm mistaken. Thank you for calling this to my attention. I'll do some checking, and I'll let you know what happens.' Well, he never did let me know what happened and I didn't realize until a good deal later that he continued to talk and write about those control, unoperated eyes as if they had been successful grafts."

Another of Summerlin's postdoctoral fellows, Dr. John Raaf, freshly arrived on a fellowship from Boston, confirmed Ninnemann's tale of misrepresentation. Raaf was culturing and transplanting parathyroid glands in rats, tiny structures in the neck astride the thyroid gland that control the exchange of calcium between bone and blood. Raaf related, "In October, about a month after I arrived in the lab, I was in the animal surgery room on the eleventh floor working on my experiments with rat parathyroid glands when Dr. Mondino was doing some corneal transplants on the rabbits. In the course of discussing what we were both doing, it came out that he was transplanting corneas to just one eye of each rabbit. I remembered that when I had first arrived in the lab the previous month, Dr. Summerlin had showed me some rabbits and had represented them as having had transplants in both eyes, and so I was quite surprised. Shortly after I talked to Dr. Mondino, I went to speak to Bill Summerlin about this and he said, 'Well, let me get in touch with Dr. Laino [Dr. Mondino's supervisor on the cornea project] and find out if that's generally true because it was my understanding that some of the rabbits had been doubly transplanted.' And later that very day—I remember we had discussed it in the morning—Dr. Summerlin came to me and said, 'I've talked to Dr. Laino and you're absolutely correct. Only one cornea per rabbit was transplanted.' I accepted this and was glad we had it straightened out and that's the last I heard about it. Bill had, as he used to put it, 'two very lovely slides' that showed transplanted corneas but it was just one eye and they had been done in Minnesota. He showed these at several meetings, I believe, and I had no reason to think there was anything wrong with that presentation.

"Whether or not you transplant corneas limbus to limbus, there has to be a scar where the sutures were put in. Dr. Summerlin had been presenting these rabbits as complete transplants so that no scarring was visible and no suture line. I recall expressing amazement that no scar was visible. But none of us who saw these animals were ophthalmologists, so I guess we just assumed that a cornea could heal in without a scar."

Despite the doubts expressed by Medawar, the poor results Ninnemann was having with his mice, and the explanation of the rabbit misunderstanding, Summerlin later in October was ebulliently optimistic in addressing a meeting of the Society of Memorial Sloan-Kettering Cancer Center. The monthly sessions of this group feature briefings by a scientist or clinician to the women who help support the hospital and research institute by holding balls and rummage sales, running its thrift shop, staging fashion shows, and the like. One of the society's mentors on the center's staff said the enchanted ladies, hearing of such startling progress in transplantation, would probably have dumped the contents of their collective purses and wallets into Summerlin's figurative hat had he asked them to support his work then and there. (The purses and wallets of the society

members contain a higher proportion of $10 and $20 bills than
do those of the average housewife.)

It wasn't that Summerlin wasn't passing the hat, but he
was passing it in the form of applications for research grants
where the hand-outs are in checks for $10,000. (Every senior
cancer researcher in the nation is expected by his or her institution to put in for one or more grants from the National Cancer
Institute, the American Cancer Society, the Damon Runyon-
Walter Winchell Cancer Fund, or one of the dozens of other
foundations whose charters include support of medical projects.)
The time seemed ripe for Summerlin to cash in on his newly
acquired fame.

Encouraged both by Good and by the "development" personnel of the cancer center, though occasionally without clearing
his applications through the proper channels, Summerlin had
applied to six groups for support between March and August of
1973. These included both the national board and the local
chapter of the American Cancer Society, the Diabetes Foundation, the Dermatology Foundation, and the Runyon Fund. None
of these were impressed enough by the urgency of funding Dr.
Summerlin's work to rate it high enough for support, though it
may be surmised that the size and supposed wealth of support
available to Memorial Sloan-Kettering may have weighed against
awards by the smaller groups.

Despite these setbacks, Good was making ample funds available to Summerlin through allocations from the big research grant
—exceeding $9 million—made by the National Cancer Institute
(NCI) to the Sloan-Kettering Institute. This award from the
budget of the National Institutes of Health, which is annually
set by the Congress out of tax revenues, was allocated by Sloan-
Kettering among its scientists and informally approved on a sum-
by-sum basis by the NCI. Thus in U.S. fiscal year 1974, which
started July 1, 1973, NCI had Summerlin down on its books for
$188,070 out of what was termed the "single-instrument grant"
to Sloan-Kettering. Of this sum, Summerlin was entitled to draw
approximately $50,000 in salary and fringe benefits.

The big annual grant to the Sloan-Kettering Institute was
being eliminated, however, in fiscal 1975, in favor of individual

and competitive project grants, and so on June 1, 1973, a sizable bundle of paper from Summerlin was delivered to the Division of Research Grants at the National Institutes of Health in Bethesda. The bulky document asked for $126,585 to support Summerlin's immunology studies for the first year and sought total funding of $629,954 over a projected five-year period. (It is the custom of the government health agency to allow another 30 to 35 per cent of the grant total as a supplement for what are termed "indirect" expenses—equipment, animal maintenance, secretarial help, etc.)

When a scientist seeks support from the nation's medical cashbox, his application is put through an exceedingly fine bureaucratic-scientific screen along the following lines. An officer of the Division of Research Grants at the NIH reads the application and pigeon-holes it for one of the eleven national institutes or, in cases of ambiguity, for two. The targets of the institutes range from broad concepts, such as "child health and human development," to specifics, such as the eye. Simultaneously, the office in the grants division sends a copy of the application to a study section of the NIH, in effect a panel of about a dozen scientists in one of about forty categories lined up roughly along medical school curricular boundaries. Summerlin's application clearly belonged to the immunobiology study section, but because of the relatively recent importance of immunologic concepts to cancer research—and probably because the applicant was employed by a cancer center—the Summerlin request was given two parents, NCI and the National Institute of Allergy and Infectious Diseases (NIAID). The closest the organ-and-disease-oriented National Institutes of Health get to immunologic disease is the classification "Allergy," now generally understood to be an illness in which one of the body's protective mechanisms is set at a self-destructively high level for normally innocuous substances such as ragweed pollen, bee venom, or penicillin. The Summerlin application would, therefore, have two chances of success. If Allergy, its primary target as decreed by the allocator, would not give it a home, Cancer was empowered to adopt the waif.

Each of the national institutes has an advisory council of outside scientists that rates grant applications forwarded as ap-

proved by the NIH study sections. The latter meet three times a
year, in January, April, and September, the results of their deliberations being sent along to the appropriately designated institute councils for their meetings about six weeks later, i.e., in
March, June, and November.

The homework of the study sections is laborious—the National
Cancer Institute alone is besieged for funds by some two thousand scientists each year. The applications to be read before
each of the three annual meetings can run to more than a
hundred. The deliberations of the study sections are as secret as
those of any club admissions committee, but NIH officials are
always ready to entertain questions from the applicant except for
who voted how. The immunobiology study section read and
discussed Summerlin's request for more than $600,000 and
decided to postpone their decision. The scientists could do this
with impeccable propriety by naming what the NIH calls a "site
committee" to visit Summerlin's lab, question him closely to
clear up any fuzzy areas, and make an estimate of his and his associates' competence to undertake the tissue-grafting studies proposed. Neither the allergy nor the cancer council could take up
the grant request in November of 1973 since it takes time to get
half a dozen professors of medicine, surgery and cell biology
who comprise a site committee to agree to meet at the same
place on the same date.

Convene the site committee did, however, on January 7, 1974,
in the Kettering Laboratory, to be shown a variety of animals in
which the organs of other creatures were said to be thriving. The
rabbits, supposedly viewing their captors through at least one
human cornea, were shown, as was a female mouse known as
"the Old Man." This brown, speckled animal had on its back a
patch of skin that had been taken from an albino mouse and
grown in tissue culture before grafting in November of 1971, according to the label on its bin. (It had received its sexually erroneous name by virtue of being grafted in the company of a
number of male mice in Summerlin's laboratory at the University
of Minnesota.)

One member of the visiting site committee was Dr. Billingham, the biologist who had collaborated with Dr. Medawar in

the classic British experiments in the 1950s. Another was Dr. Matthew D. Scharff, professor of cell biology at the Albert Einstein College of Medicine, Yeshiva University, in the Bronx. Dr. Scharff remembers that the group was not unimpressed by what they saw and were told by Dr. Summerlin, but he also recalls disquieting doubts that led to disagreement. All were aware of the enormous difficulties involved in interpreting the results of tissue culture, chief among these being identification of ownership of cells after grafting. The visibility of a scar offers ready evidence that even when one replaces one's own tissue in the normal way, the skin doesn't look exactly like what it replaced.

The nagging doubts of the site committee were still shared to a degree by the Sloan-Kettering director, Good. Now, in January 1974, Good wrote a note to his associate suggesting that he proceed with care and caution and get his research data in good order before undertaking further advanced experiments. During this period, too, Ninnemann was trying to learn from Summerlin why his (Ninnemann's) mouse grafts were so uniformly unsuccessful, and Laino wrote a letter to Summerlin that effectively demolished the latter's corneal transplantation claims: "A total of about 20 rabbits have been grafted with human donor material that was first passed through tissue culture. It appears that no appreciable difference in acceptance or rejection time occurs when these eyes are compared to others grafted directly into recipients without having first been passed through tissue culture. They both fail at about the same time."

Time, indeed, seemed to be running out on the young dermatologist and on his defiance of the immunologic dogmas of incompatible grafts so carefully defined by Medawar. When the NIH immunobiology study section convened later in January, the scientists voted not to approve Summerlin's work for funding by either the allergy or the cancer institutes. The site committee had evidently not been sufficiently impressed. This rejection, however, was not final. The advisory councils for the allergy or the cancer institutes would review the decision at their March sessions and could, if they so chose, ask the immunobiology section to reconsider its verdict.

Early in March 1974, Summerlin again demonstrated his gift

for convincing others that he was on to something important. He gave a talk in Boston that happened to be attended by one of the members of the advisory council for the National Cancer Institute. The researcher, who insists on anonymity, was so enthusiastic about what he heard that later in the month he talked the cancer council into recommending reconsideration of Summerlin's grant request by the immunobiology study section.

By this time, though, Ninnemann had gone to Good in a mood of deep chagrin. He asked his chief mentor if it would not be proper now to publish to the scientific community his negative results based on experiments with literally hundreds of mice. Good, aware of the mounting chorus of nays from other research centers, readily agreed. The problem was that, as chief of Ninnemann's section, Summerlin's name would have to appear as a coauthor of a report that refuted his own research.

There matters stood on the morning when Bill Summerlin was offered crepes and champagne for breakfast by his secretaries, and when he set forth across East Sixty-eighth Street carrying his most recently transplanted mice, the white animals with the gray grafts.

4

NEW FACES AND AN OLD GUARD

IT WASN'T JUST the arrival of the charming dermatologist with his rapid-fire claims of monumental progress in
transplantation that was shaking the conservative cancer center
on New York's ultraestablishment East Side. Even if William
Summerlin had taken his mice elsewhere, Robert Good would
have found incipient rebellion in the Sloan-Kettering laboratories when he came to Manhattan at the beginning of 1973 with

Minnesota, and his clearly stated intention of reorganizing
the troubled cancer research center.

No stabilized authority could smooth his way, either. Good's
boss as president of the over-all authority, the Memorial Sloan-
Kettering Cancer Center, had also just been appointed. Dr. Lewis
Thomas, like Good an immunologist, had been recruited by
the center's board from Yale University School of Medicine
where he had been dean, and he was more used to the quiet
vineyards of academia and research than to exacting some measure of obedience from a cageful of tigers (the senior surgeons of
Memorial Hospital) and lions (the senior research staff of Sloan-
Kettering Institute). The latter were immediately set to growling
by the elevation by Good of another young man, Dr. Lloyd
Old, as his second in command. They were also complaining that
their academic faculty prerogatives had been flouted with un-
precedented chutzpah by Good's appointments of his protégés
from Minnesota to the equivalent ranks of professors and associate professors without a vote by the members of the institute.

The growing chorus of protest, still, in early 1974, whirling
around the heads of Thomas and Good had its origins years before, with the formation of the institute and the optimistic approach to cancer control that was prevalent in the 1940s.

At the end of World War II, new chemical winds were stirring
in medicine. Cannily engineered molecules had protected allied
servicemen and women from malaria, albeit with a little yellow
added to their skin. Sir Alexander Fleming's chance observation
of a culture in a Petri dish had led to the mass production of a
historically effective drug, penicillin, which had drastically cut
the mortality from infection traditional for soldiers in the field
hit by odd shards of metal. If drugs could perform these wonders, could they not overcome cancer as well?

By 1945 the two major weapons against tumors—surgery
and radiation—were, if not well understood, at least widely used.
And in Coley's toxin long before World War II there had been
an adumbration of immune therapy. There had also been an hor-
rendous accident in Naples during World War II when Axis
forces blew up an American ship loaded to the gunwales with
mustard gas. A few observant physicians called upon to treat

sailors blown into the harbor, at that point a dilute soup of toxic nitrogen mustard, noticed that many of their patients died of bone-marrow poisoning—that is, of anemia and lack of white blood cells and platelets made in marrow—and not of burns or sea-water inhalation. This observation led some acute cancer researchers to speculate that nitrogen mustard could be used to treat leukemia, a blood cancer characterized by excessive production of immature white cells. Perhaps, they speculated, it could be used against other tumors as well. Though this observation was not to lead to mankind's first effective cancer drug until several years later, something was astir comparable to the impact of Hitler's V-2 rockets from Peenemunde on postwar aircraft engines and space flight.

The mover and shaker who noticed such hints was an automotive engineer, Charles F. Kettering of General Motors. In 1945 he and his boss Alfred P. Sloan, Jr., were encouraged to conceive the idea of a new institute devoted to cancer research. They recruited other wealthy business men, notably Frank Howard, research and engineering chief of Standard Oil (New Jersey) to put their research center in proximity to Memorial Hospital, the nation's first cancer hospital, founded on Manhattan's Upper West side in 1884 and relocated to East Sixty-eighth Street in 1939. Research at Memorial had been established after the daughter of James Douglas, a metallurgist and geologist, but originally trained as a physician, succumbed to breast cancer in 1910. Douglas, a Scots-educated Canadian of immense wealth, curiosity, and learning gave Memorial's research director, the redoubtable and fiercely parsimonious pathologist Dr. James Ewing, a total of $600,000, derived from copper mining, mainly to conduct research into the value of new radiation therapy. In fact, Douglas, with the help of the United States Government and a Philadelphia philanthropist, established, before World War I, what might be considered the predecessor of the Atomic Energy Commission. The National Radium Institute mined carnotite in Colorado and managed to extract from it 8.5 grams of radium; up to that time the entire American supply of the radioactive element amounted to only 1.3 grams. According to Memorial Hospital's official biographer, Hearst reporter Bob Considine,

"When the radium was divided among the partners in 1917, Douglas gave his share, 3.75 grams, to Memorial."

The radiation laboratory donated by Douglas opened that same year, 1917. Far more important in the history of Memorial's cancer research effort, however, was a gift of $250,000 in 1926 for the purchase of more radium and for new investigations from Edward S. Harkness, the philanthropic son of a partner of John D. Rockefeller. It was from Harkness's association with the oil magnate's son, John D. Rockefeller, Jr., that both the Rockefeller family's and Jersey Standard's (now Exxon) abiding support for the hospital stemmed. The junior Rockefeller was advised by his research beneficiaries at the Rockefeller Institute (now University) to support Dr. Ewing. Starting in 1927, the father of the current board chairman of the cancer center, Laurance Rockefeller, gave $60,000 a year for clinical and basic research and added other moneys with a liberal hand as they were needed.

Once the Rockefeller family had adopted Memorial, it was virtually certain that other corporate philanthropists would lend a hand. Among these were General Electric and the Donner family and General Motors through Messrs. Sloan and Kettering.*

The first director of the institute was Dr. Cornelius Packard ("Dusty") Rhoads, formerly of the Rockefeller Institute and director of Memorial Hospital as successor to Ewing, who had

---

* In 1974 the list of officers of the center began as follows: Laurance Rockefeller (Rockefeller Brothers Fund), chairman of the board; Benno C. Schmidt (J. H. Whitney & Company), vice-chairman; James B. Fisk (Bell Laboratories), vice-chairman; Dr. Lewis Thomas, president; William Rockefeller (Shearman & Sterling), secretary; James H. Wickersham (Morgan Guaranty Trust Company), treasurer. Among the non-scientific board members were: Christopher J. Elkus (Morgan Guaranty Trust Company); Peter O. Crisp (Rockefeller Family & Associates); Harold W. Fisher (Exxon); Clifton C. Garvin, Jr. (Exxon); James D. Landauer (his own company); Richard D. Lombard (Dominick Management Corporation); Malcolm McLean (McLean Industries); Elmore C. Patterson (Morgan Guaranty Trust Company); James D. Robinson III (American Express); H. Virgil Sherrill (Shields & Company); Robert E. Strawbridge (Strawbridge & Clothier, of Philadelphia); Carl W. Timpson, Jr. (Pershing & Company); and Harper Woodward (Rockefeller Family & Associates).

died of bladder cancer in 1943. Dr. Rhoads's approach to funding was as informal as his supervision of his scientists. With excellent contacts in Washington, he got federal dollars as easily as a talented fly fisherman takes trout, finding them in pools where others had not thought to try. The United States cancer program made its first heavy commitment in antitumor drug screening to the Sloan-Kettering Institute under Dr. Rhoads in the early 1950s.

The Naples mustard-gas disaster had now given rise to a series of so-called "nitrogen mustard drugs" that had apparent antitumor effects. In Boston the late Dr. Sidney Farber had for the first time in human history demonstrated life prolongation in acute leukemia of children with a new kind of cancer chemotherapy. Amethopterin, or methotrexate, as it is now termed, was not an antibiotic, not a substance made by a micro-organism as was penicillin to kill another micro-organism. The compound Dr. Farber gave to the dying children in Boston in the late 1940s was, so to speak, engineered to interfere with the normal reproductive processes of cells. An antimetabolite, it took the place of another chemical in a vital reproductive process but then jammed the mechanism.

As a result of this modest success with childhood leukemia—and the progress was measured in months of added survival instead of years as is the case today—the country embarked upon a vast program of synthesizing and screening a wide variety of compounds, antibiotics as well as a variety of purine and pyrimidine relatives, since the two latter classes of chemicals are end products or intermediates in many vital cell transactions.

Today's older echelon of Sloan-Kettering researchers at that time formed the nub of the country's cancer drug screening effort. There were chemists like George Brown and Jack Fox and the Japanese Kanematsu Sugiura (who had had to do his work under house arrest during World War II); biochemists like C. Chester Stock, Aaron Bendich and M. Earl Balis; pharmacologists like Frederick Philips; and drug-oriented clinicians like Dr. Joseph Burchenal and the late Dr. David Karnofsky, who had worked on mustard gases, their effects and their antidotes, for the military during the war.

Coupled with the job of making and testing hundreds of compounds that might arrest cancers was the contrasting task of finding chemicals that, inhaled or eaten by rats or mice or guinea pigs or painted on their shaven skin, would induce cancers that could then serve to indicate drug effects on human tumors. It was as a part of this effort that Sloan-Kettering internist, Dr. Ernest Wynder, who now heads his own research institute, found in the mid-1950s that benzpyrene extracted from cigarette smoke would produce cancer when painted on the skin of mice.

In two decades of laborious work, supplemented by the efforts of a number of major pharmaceutical houses and by groups in other cancer centers, there have emerged only about a dozen effective antitumor drugs. These, however, attack cells in a number of different ways and are only now, in teams of three and four and in alternating sequences, beginning to produce hopeful results in some forms of cancer. The Sloan-Kettering evaluators—and there were many more than are mentioned above—had a hand in proving the efficacy of most of the antitumor drugs in standard use today, but they did not actually discover any of the compounds, and, by and large, their work has gone largely unrecognized vis-à-vis prizes, fame, or other scientific emoluments. (One exception was the sharing of a Lasker award by Burchenal in 1972.)

These indefatigable investigators did, however, have one advantage over their brethren sweating out the search for cancer drugs in other laboratories. They did not have to stop working periodically to concoct an appeal for funding from the National Cancer Institute or the foundations. The NIH in Maryland had recognized that an effort of the scope and longevity needed to procure effective antitumor agents could not be carried on piecemeal with grants that had to be renewed each year. So the federal cancer experts turned to the device so successfully used for other purposes by the Pentagon and other government agencies where procurement also involved research and development: The federal cancer experts let out contracts to drug houses like Upjohn, Pfizer, and Lilly to make and test new compounds and they contracted with Rhoads at Sloan-Kettering to take the next more sophisticated steps in the screening of these agents and in making additional ones. Such large contracts became, in effect, the precedent for the unique funding arrangement of the National Institutes of Health with Sloan-Kettering.

Rhoads died in 1959 and was replaced in 1960 by another former Rockefeller Institute scientist, a specialist in viral diseases whose style was the antithesis of Rhoads's open and almost flamboyant approach to funding, spending, and publicity. Dr. Frank Horsfall was a shy, somewhat aloof scientist who held the firm conviction that the less said about cancer research and any progress therein, the better. It was under Dr. Horsfall, in 1965, that the single-instrument grant from the National Cancer Institute to Sloan-Kettering came to fruition. At the time, Sloan-Kettering scientists were working under more than fifty separate grants from the federal agency, which was then headed by Dr. Kenneth Endicott. Horsfall and Endicott agreed that entirely too much time was being spent by talented researchers in shuffling lengthy grant applications down to Bethesda and revising them endlessly to conform with some bureaucratic whim. Why not have Sloan-Kettering itself be the applicant, subsuming in one application projects for radiation therapy research, surgical innovations, viral causation studies, drug screening, and so forth? The individual investigators would then report periodically to their own chiefs and be allocated funds from the single large grant.

The deal was made, but not without some audible gripes from other cancer centers and other scientists involved in work on tumors. The agreement stipulated that Sloan-Kettering would set an annual budget based on old and new projects and that 47.3 per cent of that budget would be supplied from NCI funds, leaving the Memorial Sloan-Kettering Cancer Center to raise the rest either from bequests, gifts, or grants from private foundations.

The first single-instrument grant in 1966 came to more than $4 million and by 1969 was over $5 million. With increasing knowledge about viruses, cell metabolism, drug action, and tumor immunology came added opportunities for broadening the research base, and Sloan-Kettering's budget swelled accordingly. In 1971, the year the Memorial Sloan-Kettering Cancer Center lost both Horsfall and its president, Richard Vanderwarker, to cancer,

the total Sloan-Kettering Institute budget had climbed to over
$12 million. By 1973 it had almost reached $15 million.

When Thomas, as president of the center, and Good, as director of the institute, arrived to take over the reins that year, both
center and institute had been operating under caretaker regimes
for almost two years. Acting president of the center was the bluff
and easygoing former Memorial Hospital comptroller, David W.
Walsh, who quite simply lacked the presence and the credentials
that Laurance Rockefeller and his board knew would be necessary to guide the center through its new career as a forward bas-
tion in the Nixonian all-out war against cancer. Likewise, Dr.
Leo Wade, a former industrial physician whom Horsfall had
chosen to bring order out of the Rhoadsian chaos, headed the
institute with more of a fussy flair for neatness and order than
any desire to shape its goals or shape up its troops. Under Wade,
a half-dozen old-timers serving as the elected vice-presidents of
the institute under the broad authority of its senate, i.e., the de-
greed professional personnel, effectively ran the place. The vice-
presidents knew that Dr. Wade, nearing retirement, might fuss
and fume over certain actions, policies, and requests, but they
were also confident that they would get their way eventually.
The tyrants, Ewing, Rhoads, Horsfall, were in their graves, and
it seemed that a quasi-academic democracy was within the
members' grasp.

Larger forces were at work, however, to frustrate them. In
1969 the then-new Nixon administration was happily swinging
its budgetary scythe through the fields of medical training and
research. Money, especially money for training young scientists
and physicians, one of Memorial Sloan-Kettering's fortes, became
as scarce as daisies in January. The cries of pain and anguish
could be heard from every medical school and medical center in
the land. The professors of surgery and medicine and radiology
and pediatrics and psychiatry had built their empires of residents and postdoctoral fellows, of laboratories and costly electronic devices, of glass washers and animal caretakers mainly
with government money. And now the federal Office of Management and the Budget, the despised OMB, was turning the handle
of the faucet in the wrong direction.

Mrs. Albert Lasker, widow of the advertising magnate and champion of larger medical research funding, renewed her efforts at parties and dinners, where she expertly mingled famous cancer researchers like Boston's Sidney Farber and famous open-heart surgeons like Houston's Michael De Bakey with influential senators and congressmen from strategic committees. But all Mary Lasker's doctors and all of her District of Columbia knights made little impact on the budget chopping that the President had set in motion.

The big New York cancer center was less hamstrung than many, but it, too, felt the pinch. Its annual report for 1970 was entitled "Year of Crisis," and the Sloan-Kettering Institute and Memorial Hospital combined to run a deficit of $2 million that had to be painfully extracted from endowment accounts. It was in the midst of this disastrous cutback that Nixon, egged on by some members of Congress, by his long-time pharmaceutical millionaire patron Elmer Holmes Bobst, by Benno Schmidt, and by the American Cancer Society, signed a bill to further the control of cancer, a Manhattan atomic project, if you will, against the country's most feared if not its most lethal disease.

In 1972, through ups and downs of presidential-congressional haggling and hassling, some large money numbers surfaced, vanished, surfaced again. For the Sloan-Kettering Institute, though, the news had to be good. If the single-instrument grant was beginning to look a little threadbare to both parties involved and encouraging, as it seemed to, a stand-pat attitude among senior researchers, rescue seemed at hand. But no sooner had the lines of authority been established in Washington and the bigger appropriations voted to the National Cancer Institute than many scientists and medical administrators who had previously objected to all that money going to one disease started organizing suitable programs which would entitle *them* to some.

In New York, Mount Sinai Medical Center was by 1970 at the brink of bankruptcy, having started a new medical school just as the money tree withered in Washington. So Mount Sinai hired a leading cancer investigator from Buffalo's Roswell Park Memorial Institute in an effort to qualify for some of the new cancer funds. Columbia Presbyterian Medical Center uptown on the

Hudson River suddenly began making headlines about cancer with its special unit for the disease. These two other centers were not alone. Partly by government design, in a move to create two dozen new centers of cancer expertise across the nation, and partly from the ingenuity born of starvation, tumor institutes were blossoming all over the country.

The largest of the nation's cancer research centers, with its trustee and vice-chairman Benno Schmidt serving as one of the President's trio of cancer advisers, the Memorial-Sloan Kettering Cancer Center now found itself competing with new cancer centers all clamoring for part of the federal money. What had seemed due by right to the nation's pre-eminent cancer enclave was now being contested, albeit in gentlemanly style, by new-comers. This scurry for cancer dollars could not have gone unnoticed at the Rockefeller Family offices, at J. H. Whitney & Company, or in other well-paneled suites to which the Memorial Sloan-Kettering search committees reported. Their ultimate choices were men with proven records—Thomas, a former Yale dean with impeccable credentials, and Good, a Minnesota professor who was judged to have as good a chance as anybody at a Nobel prize and whose prowess as a fund raiser was second to none.

With Good's appointment as director of the Sloan-Kettering Institute, Laurance Rockefeller, Benno Schmidt, and their board of trustees bypassed the old-guard vice-presidents and buried their power under a fund-raising machine oiled by a philosophy closely linked to that of the founding fathers of the Sloan-Kettering Institute.

Messrs. Sloan and Kettering had planned their research enclave not as an ivory tower but as a patient-oriented, pragmatic push against cancer. Had they known him, Robert Good would have been their ideal choice for leader. "If you listen to him, the patient will teach you," Good preaches. This was a far cry from the pure research endorsed by Horsfall and the senior staffers of the institute. The contest between results for survival's sake and data for the sake of knowledge had been decided in the board room. If the nation was to be mobilized and its tax moneys spent to conquer cancer, what was wanted, the board decreed, were the results that Good implied, if he did not actually promise.

One of the first exhibitions of Good's power was his appointment of William Summerlin as a full member of the Sloan-Kettering Institute. Good simply ignored the institute's tradition by which nominations for the various ranks—member, associate member, research associate, etc.—were cleared by an advisory committee of scientists and by the half-dozen vice-presidents of the institute and then submitted to the board of trustees for approval. Good named his Minnesota people to the levels he felt they should occupy, and the board rubber-stamped them.

Later, chided about Summerlin's elevation, Good explained that his protégé had had "other lucrative offers" and that the membership, as well as the $50,000 annual salary (including benefits), had been necessary to get him to come to New York. Later, too, Summerlin partly confirmed this while denying it. He said, "I didn't feel like I'd completed my work or interaction with Bob Good and I was at a critical crossroads where I had to decide was I going to New York with Bob Good or go somewhere else. I've been told it's been said that I had a lot of offers from universities around the country. That's simply not so. I told Bob that the Mayo Clinic wanted me to come down there on their staff. That was very close by and I knew some people down there [Rochester, Minnesota]. . . . And the only other place I visited at all—even considered—was Duke. I had an offer of an associate professorship there. But almost from the outset I decided that I was going to go to New York and I told him that. So it wasn't as if I had been trying to bargain one place against the other and get some one-upmanship. That's just simply not the case. I committed myself to coming with him, and the reason had nothing to do with the war on cancer or Sloan-Kettering . . . but because of Bob Good. In retrospect, I have to plead guilty to an overdose of hero worship. You know, I felt very close to this man. Regrettably, it wasn't mutual, as it turned out."

In another early move, Good appointed Lloyd Old, a fellow immunologist and a long-term Sloan-Kettering hand as his administrative deputy, i.e., as a vice-president and associate director of the institute. (The scientist vice-presidents had been asked to submit their resignations before Good's official arrival date, January 1, 1973, and had duly tendered them.) Old, a tall, boyish bachelor of matchless unease, brilliant immunologic competence, and no discernible human foibles except pride, had been for a decade the member of the institute most irritating to the senior members. They could not put him down as a newcomer. They could not fault his scientific competence. His publications were cited in the best circles and his lectures were crystalline discourses that would draw a packed house at any medical institution in the nation.

The reaction of the senior researchers to Old was purely visceral. He just didn't feel right to men and women who had sweated so long to attain what seemed to come easily to this bright young man not even forty.

It is not easy for those outside of science to recognize the prejudices that hide beneath the professed objectivity of white coats. Had Good chosen Dr. Andrew Ivy, promoter of the discredited cancer drug, krebiozen, as his deputy, the reaction of some members could not have been more categorically negative.

Finally, there was the immunologic concept of cancer itself, one that conceded grudgingly a role for radiation and chemotherapy after the surgeons had done what they could or thrown up their scalpels in well-concealed despair and frustration. A handful of clinicians at Memorial were gingerly attempting immunotherapy and immunologic gauging of the cancer patient's ability to recognize his or her tumor cells as foreigners and reject them, as the dogma dictated for cells with strange chemical markings etched upon them. And out there in other research laboratories, both in the United States and abroad, dark hints were being voiced that the drugs that poisoned bone marrow along with the tumor cells and thus reduced the body's competence to fight invaders might be counterproductive in a devastating way. The same obtained for many forms of radiation therapy.

Good came to the Sloan-Kettering Institute with the conviction that a complete understanding of the human immune system would lead to progress in cancer control. It was not to be expected that scientists and physicians who had devoted most of their working lives to battling the surgeons inch by painful inch to make a niche for drug treatment before the patient lapsed into a final coma would welcome this. Typical was the reaction of one senior chemotherapist at the institute when asked whether treatment to bolster the patient's immune system might not already be a first line of treatment for malignant melanoma, the lethal skin cancer that quickly invades the viscera, spreads like a prairie fire, and kills quickly. "Rubbish," said the drug-oriented physician.

Rubbish or not, the Australian Nobel laureate Dr. MacFarlane Burnet had examined all the evidences available in the 1950s and had pieced together a coherent theory of organisms, including humans, identifying "self" and distinguishing "self" from "nonself," and the importance of their doing so. A few years later, in the 1960s, Burnet and Thomas, then at New York University, proposed that the immune system was not only useful against true invaders but also mounted its attack against any of the body's own cells that started to act strangely by making proteins (antigens, by definition) that were detected as foreign by its presumed surveillance system. Such cells, as we have seen, would include tumor cells.

Cancer thus might be a special case of malignant immunologic tolerance, one that put the host in dire jeopardy. There are a number of possible clues that cancer researchers are now puzzling over. Among them: the tumor manages, so to speak, to hide its special antigens, its foreignness, from the defensive force of white cells. Or perhaps the white cells coat the tumor with ineffective antibody that serves only to conceal it or protect it against lymphocyte assault. Or the attacking white cells are rendered ineffective by some feature of the cancer, or else at a certain stage there are simply not enough of them to control the situation, implying that when the tumor was very, very young and small it might have escaped detection by white cells assigned a putative surveillance role. (Nobody has yet seen a one- or two- or four-celled cancer just starting its destructive rampage in a patient.)

In any case, most immunologists concerned about cancer, and Good is among their number, now believe that in many in-

stances cancer victims are, in fact, suffering from some immunologic deficit that disables the lymphocyte system in one of
its aspects. Thus the first tumor cells with the chemical mark of
Cain upon them, are not destroyed forthwith but are tolerated
until they have become so numerous that the host defenses are
overwhelmed. Evidence leading to this conclusion has grown
stronger ever since Dr. Ludwik Gross found he could immunize
a mouse against tumor from a twin by injecting the malignant
cells and then removing them surgically. He discovered in the
1950s that he could not put in for the second go-round just any
sized tumor he wished. With tumors above a certain size, even
the delayed hypersensitivity reaction—the amplified production
of special tumor-killer cells—would not be enough to save the
life of the mouse recipient.

Another bit of evidence comes from infants born with an
inherited defect in their immune system attributable to a defective chromosome. The specific defect is exceedingly rare and is
known as ataxia-telangiectasia. Babies with this form of congenital abnormality are now known to suffer a much higher incidence of cancer early in life. So are children with Bloom's
syndrome, a condition in which genetic material is arbitrarily
exchanged among chromosomes in somatic cells, but in the latter
case, no immune deficiency has yet been identified.

Finally, just in the last few years, a group of statisticians at the
University of Minnesota, under the urging of Good, have been
maintaining a cancer registry enrolling kidney-transplant patients. Such patients must receive for months and years drugs
that depress their white cell defenses. The body does not quickly
give up on its attempts to reject a grafted kidney that comes
from anyone other than an identical twin. Such transplant recipients now usually live five to ten years and more, and an unusually high percentage of them have developed cancer. The evidence points to the drug-induced immune suppression as a
critical factor in the susceptibility to malignancy.

It was in pursuit of additional evidence to support the theory
that cancer patients are immunologically deficient that a member
of the Sloan-Kettering Institute got into trouble in the 1960s. To
Dr. Chester Southam must go the credit for the first exhaustive

investigation of the immune capacity of human beings, but in 1965, two years after his experiments, it cost him his license to practice medicine in the state of New York. Dr. Southam, a tall, cool physician asked for and received permission from a group of dying cancer patients to put patches of other people's skin on their bodies.

If the previous animal work by other researchers meant anything at all, these cancer patients should reject transplants more slowly than a burned or ulcerated patient would. Southam was gratified to find that this was the case. The lymphocytes of cancer victims were less efficient than those of normal people. But for medical scientists the key word is "control." A control, be it human or animal, is the specimen that has all of the characteristics of the diseased except the one that the experimenter is interested in. Cancer patients are, by and large, older people. They tend to suffer heart disease, diabetes, hardening of the arteries, and other conditions that afflict the aged. Since nobody had ever systematically grafted the skin of others onto a group of such patients, it was at least questionable whether age itself or one of its concomitant tissue failures might slow down transplant rejection. Furthermore, the laws of statistics would insist on a large number of controls. Otherwise, chance might play a role, and skin from a genetically compatible person might be grafted and survive long enough to skew the results of the experiment.

Southam decided to give himself the best chance available to prove his case. Cancer cells from a stranger would bear not only the individual, transplantation antigens but also the so-called tumor antigens, thus increasing the odds for rejection. Obviously, the place to go to find aged and infirm but otherwise normal people would be a hospital that catered to their needs. The controls would have to be old and sick but not dying of some identifiable disease. Their lymphocytes, should, theoretically, be both vigorous and competent and, if Southam's assumptions were correct, they would promptly destroy grafted tumor tissue.

So Southam approached young doctors at the Jewish Hospital for Chronic Disease in Brooklyn and asked if he could seek the co-operation of some of their aged patients. Young doctors fresh out of medical school are thoroughly imbued with respect for experimental medicine. In the long run, that is how they learn what they learn.

Informed consent has come to be a keystone of medicine and medical research. Before the surgeon operates, the hospital, whose operating suite he uses, has obtained from the patient a signed statement that he or she knows what is to be done, appreciates the risks, and does not hold anyone responsible for subsequent mistakes. While this does not prevent the patient in whose stomach a sponge or bit of gauze has been left inadvertently from suing, it makes hospital administrators more comfortable and helps them to sleep.

But informed consent, for Southam, would involve use of the dreadful word "cancer." If he told the old and institutionalized people that they were to receive a minute graft of tumor, most of them would have said, "No, thank you." So he solved the problem by not telling them. All they ever knew was that a small incision would be made in their arms and some cells put there to grow and, presumably, be rejected. That turned out to be the case in every instance. And the rejection was speedy enough to confirm Southam's hypothesis. It wasn't just age and debility that crippled people's immune systems. It had something to do with having cancer.

The trouble was that one of the young doctors at the home did not agree with Southam's definition of "informed consent," and he later brought the experiment to the attention of the authorities, namely, the New York State Board of Regents, whose function it is to license physicians. Though the regents recognized the importance of Southam's experiment, they agreed with the young doctor that the patients had not been fully and properly informed about the test in which they had served as guinea pigs. Southam's license to practice medicine was eventually—in December 1965—suspended, and five years later he left the state to accept a professional post at Jefferson Medical College in Philadelphia.

The subject of well-matched organ donors and recipients led in the early 1960s to some fruitful attempts to keep human lymphocytes alive in culture. The reasoning of the pioneers in this endeavor, Dr. Fritz Bach and Dr. Kurt Hirschhorn, both then at

New York University School of Medicine, was that if these were the cells that accomplished the destruction of an incompatible graft, one might, by taking samples of these white cells from prospective organ donors and recipients and putting them together to grow in dishes or test tubes, be able to ascertain the degree of incompatibility of the two people, donor and recipient, before taking the relatively irrevocable step of cutting a kidney out of one and sewing it into the other.

Just after the turn of the century, when Dr. Karl Landsteiner solved the problem of blood transfusion by determining the ABO group of red-cell antigens and providing physicians with a means of testing for their presence (he also collaborated in the finding of the Rh factor in 1940), it became apparent that varying loci on the chromosomes differentiated one person from another not only by height, hair and eye color, skin pigmentation, skin-ridge patterns, and so forth, but also by invisible markers that are now termed "transplantation antigens." The function of these markers seems to be to give the body its defensive sense of selfness. These tissue markers are not all determined by sequences of nucleotides in the DNA at one locus or place on a single chromosome but are scattered throughout our genetic endowment.

However, one locus called "HLA-1" has now been studied exhaustively and appears to be the strongest determinant for antigens that cause rejection in incompatible transplants. At the moment, nobody knows in which of our forty-six chromosomes this locus lies. Much less can anyone read the nucleotide code to ascertain which of two siblings, for example, would be a better kidney donor for a third needing a transplant.

Surgeons now get around this problem by having immunologists check up on the literally dozens of antigens dictated by the HLA-1 chromosomal region involved. This recondite form of preoperative consultation involves obtaining antigens—often from women who have born a lot of children—and then systematically checking the donor's serum for the presence or absence of antigens that are present in the blood of the patient needing the transplant. Because of the Mendelian genetic laws, the chances of obtaining a good match for HLA-1 markers is far bet-

ter among family members than among donors and recipients
who are unrelated.

In 1963 Hirschhorn and Bach decided to grow human lymphocytes in vitro and then challenge them wtih lymphocytes from
another patient or volunteer. Using various biochemical techniques, they thought they might be able more simply to detect
degrees of sameness or foreignness by the responses of the cells
to each other. This worked out, to a degree, and is in clinical
transplantation use to this day. However, Bach and Hirschhorn
had to assume that the act of culturing the white blood cells outside the body would not drastically change their antigens or
their ability to recognize foreign antigens. In other words, a cultured lymphocyte had to be assumed both to display its human
owner's antigenic flag and to recognize the pirate ensign of
another person. They did not and could not know whether recognition or action, as evidenced by a rapid change in the lymphocyte, a measurable rise in its metabolic activity was or was not
taking place in the same cell or whether recognition of strangeness was the function of one type and change and attack the
function of another.

Both Hirschhorn and Bach have, in subsequent years and
among other projects, been trying to refine their so-called "mixed
lymphocyte test" for tissue-graft compatibility. So has Dr. Paul I.
Terasaki, immunologist in the Department of Surgery of the
University of California. It was Terasaki who reported just a
month after Summerlin's suspension at Sloan-Kettering, the only
evidence to surface thus far from an expert immunologist that,
as Summerlin was claiming, some important changes took place in
very immunologically sophisticated cells when they were grown
for a period in culture.

The article appeared in the magazine *Science* for April 26,
1974, and Terasaki was saying that lymphocytes from one
human being, taken from a vein and separated from the other
blood components, then grown in culture for four days, lost their
ability to stimulate lymphocytes from a second person that were
added to their dish. The individual donors involved had been
specially selected for their incompatibility, and when the second
batch of lymphocytes were added to the first, they should have

responded with a burst of metabolic activity upon meeting at close range cells with, to them, strange chemical traits. But they didn't, Terasaki reported. So far as he could tell—and Terasaki is acknowledged to be a superior craftsman in the art of tissue matching—the original lymphocytes still had their identifying antigens.

This finding, together with other work leads some immunologists, including Good, to take Summerlin's claims seriously. Since the revelation that Summerlin had colored the skins of his mice, however, Good is inclined to advance what he calls "trivial" explanations for the graft prolongations that were occasionally seen with the Summerlin skin and organ cultures. By "trivial," a scientist means only that the reasons would not involve any major challenge to a basic dogma such as that of Burnett and Medawar.

"When I studied Summerlin's cultured grafts," Good related, "there were several things I noticed as a pathologist. First, there was the loss of passenger [patrolling] leukocytes. Then, when I looked at the blood vessels, I found that the endothelial cells that normally line them weren't present but that the basement membrane of the arterioles and venules remained intact. It seemed to me quite likely after grafting that tissue in the new host, re-establishment of circulation would be possible using those channels but with endothelial repopulation by the host's cells. Now there would be loss of another major target of immune rejection, the endothelial or lining cells of the blood vessels. And the final thing that I noticed was that the graft surface was reduced to a single or at most a double layer of cells instead of the usual seven layers, thus again reducing the target of white cell rejection."

The part of Good's explanation that involves patrolling leukocytes would also involve the following hypothesis: Suppose some observant white cells—lymphocytes, perhaps—are always wandering around in the skin looking for some invader, be it venom from a bee sting or tetanus clostridium bacteria borne on the point of a shard of glass on a beach or a nail in a board from an old barn. Suppose that such patrolling cells bear more obvious markers of their ownership, their "selfness," if you will, than the epithelial cells that lay down the protein fibers that make up our naked overcoat. Perhaps the act of cutting out a skin sample and culturing it might not be as inimical to the skin cells as it is to the guardian white cells. In a week or two, the last of the lymphocytes might die off, leaving fewer antigenic skin units behind. A delayed graft might then survive longer, with the recipient's white cells less able to perceive the foreigners.

An attractive theory but one that was obviously called into question by Terasaki's findings. Faced with a situation in which lymphocytes were not passengers but the only cell types present at all, the Californian still has to explain the loss of chemical identity as evidenced by the unresponsiveness of the stranger lymphocytes added to the "natives" in the dish.

The scientist's job, never discussed in the pages of the slick magazines, in time-starved television programs, or in the newspapers, all of which deal in supposedly established "facts," is to imagine an explanation for an observed phenomenon. If the hypothesis, the proposed explanation, is appealing, the next task is to think of some way of testing it that is as far removed as possible from the conditions of the original observation.

The problem is not just to come up with a surprising set of data but to use intelligence and experience in the broadest way possible to offer an explanation for the data that will apply to other data and that will elucidate happenings for which there has been no previous explanation. Every scientist builds on information developed by those who worked before him. The successful scientist develops a totally new way of looking at some of the information he inherited.

And so Paul Terasaki suggested in the nation's most widely read general science magazine a further subdivision of lymphocytes. Unknown to observers, he speculated, the smallest of white blood cells might be further subdivided into those with enhanced stimulatory or "this-is-me" characteristics and more self-effacing, and, perhaps, more aggressive units. Presumably the more demonstrative lymphocytes are lost in culture.

Hirschhorn, asked about this phenomenon, will say only that he thinks "something is happening in culture." Professors of genetics and pediatrics are not normally outspoken in explaining other researchers' findings. However, Hirschhorn is not inclined to bury Summerlin's observations. He says, "Lymphocytes may be amplifiers of antigenic reactions only when they are in the presence of other cells that they can recruit."

Terasaki found, paradoxically, that the cultured human lymphocytes that had seemingly lost some of their identifying markers had not lost their ability to respond to carefully calibrated challenges with certain plant-derived substances and foreign cells known to elicit reactions from lymphocytes. Perhaps the expression of cell surface markers was depressed, Terasaki suggested. And Hirschhorn hazarded that some amplifiers of cellular rejection might be inhibited.

The action in lymphocyte, tissue-typing culture is duplicated in cancer-antigen immunologic research. Researchers add lymphocytes taken from the patient to his or her own cancer cells in glass and watch for destructive processes. They also have more sophisticated means of gauging the patient's ability to fight and destroy cancer cells.

But the immunologic cancer fighters labor under a heavy handicap. They cannot try their new weapon until surgeons, radiologists, and chemotherapists have given up. By that time, whatever remnants of immune competence the patient might have had have been severely depleted. Despite the lip service paid in cancer centers to the "multidisciplinary attack on cancer," it is generally accepted in all medical centers that the surgeons get the first try at curing the patient. The scalpel is, after all, the original weapon against the disease, and the immunologists are now in fairly general agreement that the body's defenses will never be vigorous enough to obliterate a big and thriving tumor that has established its own blood supply and consists of billions of atavistic cells.

Both radiation therapy with today's high-voltage equipment and chemotherapy with drugs that are most inimical to rapidly proliferating cells have deleterious effects on the immune system. So the primacy of the radiologist and the chemotherapist cannot but prejudice the later efforts of the immunologist. Still, in both Europe and the United States there is growing evidence that after drugs have reduced the number of leukemic cells in the blood down to a few million, treatment with an agent that stimulates the immune system can play an important role in eliminating the rest. The only other form of cancer in which immune therapy, that is, therapy with relatively innocuous bacteria or chemicals that rouse the white cell defense system, has proven effective is melanoma. The results in that malignancy, however, have been limited to lesions on the skin. Once the disease has invaded the viscera, it appears to be beyond the reach of the stimulated natural immune defense.

The immunologists, however, are far from conceding defeat. For one thing, they are proselytizing surgeons, basing their arguments on the French leukemia experience, to let them use immune therapy postoperatively when the surgeon has good evidence that he hasn't been able to clean out all of the tumor and can thus expect recurrence or metastasis (spread to another site) in the near future. Instead of strong drugs that depress the bone marrow, nauseate the patient, and cause his or her hair to fall out, the immune therapist injects living bacteria, either a strain known as Corynebacterium parvum or the bacillus Calmette-Guérin (BCG) that is employed in ghetto areas to immunize children against tuberculosis. (While BCG is no more closely related to the bacillus of tuberculosis than the cowpox organism is to the smallpox virus, it can cause severe illness in certain patients, even to the point where an antituberculosis drug may be called for to cancel out the effects of the treatment.)

The immunologists hope that their less toxic—though not innocuous—materials may soften the resistance that surgeons have shown to immediate postoperative treatment that makes the patient uncomfortable even though possibly saving his or her life. Then, too, the immunologists are teaming up with chemotherapists so that their different anticancer agents can be given simultaneously. In their methods of preparing immunity-stimulants, in their dosage schedule, and in their timing, in combination with other forms of treatment, the immunotherapists still have a great deal to learn. And cancer has a remarkable ability to stir dissension and rivalry among physicians.

If a patient is laid low by pneumonia, foci of infection and infiltration of the lungs will be readily visible on X-ray plates. If the drug given to the patient is effective, the opacity in the lungs will clear up. If the patient is suffering from septicemia—the invasion of the bloodstream by toxic bacteria or viruses—the doctor can take blood samples, grow them in agar, and easily determine the benefits of his treatment.

Such is not the case with cancer after surgery. Though there is one immunologic test—for the so-called "carcinoembryonic antigen"—that may well reveal recurrence of cancer of the gastrointestinal system, it is normally the cancer the physician cannot readily detect that kills his patient. The surgeon often removes the primary tumor and sends his patient home, only to have him return a few months later with multiple metastases in inaccessible areas. Worse, the sophisticated surgeon will suspect that he may have had a hand in seeding the savage cells into the adjacent lymph channels and blood vessels at the operating table.

The radiologist, likewise, knows that his destructive beam must often penetrate healthy tissue to reach its tumor goal. He can only do his best to minimize the risks by minute dosimetric calculations to determine correct beam direction and voltage. As has been mentioned, the chemotherapist, too, spends much of his time monitoring the untoward effects his drugs produce. They can reduce platelet numbers and produce fatal hemorrhage. They can damage the heart or the lungs. They can practically eliminate the white cells, thus leaving the patient open to a lethal infection from germs always present in the hospital setting.

All three specialists face a trade-off situation in which they hope they can kill enough tumor cells without fatally compromising the patient's ability to survive.

In such a situation, physicians perforce must turn to statistics. A patient who is cured of pneumonia or septicemia is freed of disease and, presumably, stands no greater risk of a recurrence than anyone else of his age. But the cancer patient, already obviously handicapped by an immune defect or some viral invasion of his genetic material or simply by his lineage, no longer stands the same chance of survival as his peers. Given this frustrating situation of therapeutic risk and built-in susceptibility, researchers have turned to mathematics. The patient who lives five years after cancer is diagnosed is termed a cure.

Into this ambiguous morass of hopes and fears and highly charged emotions comes the immunologist with his new, untried theories, his toxins and other biologicals and his openly voiced suspicion that much of the cancer therapy of the past twenty-five or thirty years has been operating on a set of false premises. Small wonder, then, that Good's arrival at Memorial Sloan-Kettering with his implied promise of immunologic progress against cancer stirred bitter recrimination in some quarters.

5

idENTiTy ANd RECOGNiTioN

IMMUNOLOGISTS LIKE Robert Good are still hard put to explain successful pregnancies, even one where there is no Rh incompatibility between husband and wife. There, emerging from the birth canal, wriggles a small, very red, and soon very noisy exception to the rules of immunologic compatibility. Roughly half the infant is a graft from its father that has "taken" for nine months in the mother and is only now, if you like, being rejected by the uterine muscles. In the meantime, it has been spared

somehow by the maternal antibodies and white cells that should
long since have destroyed it because of the father's varied array
of antigens with which it was endowed at conception.

Here is how Dr. Barbara Jacobs and Dr. Delta Uphoff described the dilemma in *Science* for August 16, 1974: "The
successful maternal-fetal relationship has been attributed to the
placenta's being a privileged site. However, the reduced responsiveness of females toward paternal antigens of their hybrid
progeny [that is, their babies] was demonstrated by Breyere and
Barrett. . . . A successful pregnancy may require a qualitative
change in phenotypic [body cell] expression of the antigenicity of
the fetus. The reduced immunogenicity (antigenicity) of the
fetus, in turn, induces a reduction in responsiveness of the
mother to the specific alloantigens [paternal antigens] of her
fetus."

The placenta, in other words, exposes the mother to dozens of
antigens—proteins and complex sugars—dictated by the father's
share of the fetus's genes. Yet only one of these possible antigens,
the Rh (from rhesus, the species of monkeys in which it was first
isolated) factor in or on red blood cells, is capable of sensitizing
a mother who is Rh negative, i.e., lacks this marker on her
erythrocytes. Even so, the blood of the first child conceived by
an Rh incompatible couple is not usually damaged by the maternal immune reaction. It is only after a pregnancy exposure to one
Rh-positive baby that therapeutic steps have to be taken to
prevent the now-sensitized mother from destroying the red cells
of her next Rh-positive fetus.

A species has a definite survival advantage if its young spend
their first defenseless weeks or months inside the mother's body.
The eggs of birds and reptiles tempt predators with an easily obtained and highly nutritious meal. But for internal maternal protection to work, the mother has to be tolerant of the antigens
produced in the fetus by its paternal genes.

Before Summerlin announced his means of seemingly mod-
ulating the very intense immune response to foreign skin,
dozens of scientists had found complex ways of changing the antigenicity of cells and the tolerance of a potential host by adding
various factors to the medium in which the donor cells were

grown. Such researches were and are of the utmost importance, bearing as they do on the immense challenges of transplantation and cancer. To understand the issues here, some history is necessary.

Readers who were taught in school about an eighteenth-century English physician, Edward Jenner, and his daring human experiment with apparently infectious and purulent material from cowpox sores, will immediately think of an immunologist as a doctor who gives shots. And, indeed, Jenner's trust in a milkmaid's observation that lasses who got cowpox didn't get smallpox laid the cornerstone of the medical specialty. For public health, the importance of Jenner's successful vaccinations, which prevented the regular ravages of a common, disfiguring, and frequently fatal infectious disease, has come in the series of later successful immunizations—against tetanus, diphtheria, whooping cough, yellow fever, influenza, measles, German measles (rubella), and, in the midst of these, the most publicized of all, Dr. Jonas Salk's killed-virus vaccine against poliomyelitis.

For modern medical science, however, the important message was about antigens, chemical compounds either common to a group of tissues or organisms—like the similar molecules displayed by the viruses of cowpox and smallpox—or else unique to the individual creature. The latter, because of the notorious troubles they have made for surgeons, are known as transplantation antigens.

Dr. Edward Boyse of the Sloan-Kettering Institute, for example, once called the author's attention to a remarkable fact: "If you grow cells from different organs or different species in the same dish, they exhibit a clannish disposition, have in a sense some mysterious territoriality comparable to a tribe of apes or wolves. But this characteristic, which shows itself as a reluctance to grow in too close proximity to the foreign cells, the 'others,' has two facets. One is organ specific, another, species specific, if you will. Curiously enough," Dr. Boyse continued, "organ compatibility seems to supersede species compatibility so that, for example, colonies of cells from the skins of rabbits and guinea pigs will grow in the same dish more tolerantly than will cells from, say, skin and liver of the same animal."

Where did this chemical sense of selfness come from? What ends does it serve? Rather early in his career Dr. Good, tracking back down the evolutionary line, found that a very primitive fish called the hagfish has an underdeveloped sense of self and seems to lack the ability to reject tissue grafted from others. This fish also lacks a thymus gland. The observation led Good to speculate that the human thymus, the puzzling little gland in the lower neck which is large in childhood and progressively shrinks as we become mature, might have something to do with the establishment of the immune system, the cells and antibodies that guard the substance recognized as self against intrusion by substances and organisms and cells recognized as strangers.

This immune system, it now turns out, is a dual one, and Good played an important role in deciphering the rough outlines of its duality. Jenner's successful vaccinations to prevent smallpox were based on the first and best known part of the system, so-called humoral immunity, in which special white blood cells that remain in a quiescent state until summoned to activity by still poorly understood messages, probably from other white blood cells, pour out particular molecules called antibodies. Each antibody is made in such a way as to be attracted to its specific antigen, the strange molecule or cluster of strange molecules that has invaded the antibody's owner, and to cling to this antigen like a Judas. At some point, still other white blood cells are attracted to the antibody and perform an enzymatic act of destruction on the interloper.

Current theory has it that this system does not in and of itself require its owner to have a thymus gland and that this system is not the first line of defense against either cancers or grafts of foreign tissue. Here again, there is vast uncertainty in immunologic circles as to why one mechanism should have been developed by animals to cope with certain kinds of challenger antigens such as viruses, pollens, venoms, and some bacteria whereas another tribe of cells, evidently closely related to those that cunningly manufacture antibody molecules, are called upon to hurl themselves bodily upon other foreigners. Among the latter are larger and more complex parasites, the bacteria that cause tuberculosis and leprosy, tissue grafts, and, in some cases, tumor cells. It is this second category of immune response that is most concerned with the issues that boiled up at Sloan-Kettering in 1974. The cells of this second category are called T-lymphocytes, and when their action is visible, as in a positive skin reaction to tuberculin, a substance containing one or more antigens of the bacillus that causes tuberculosis, it is termed a "delayed hypersensitivity reaction."

The tuberculin test is probably the best way to outline this defense mode. A person may have had tuberculosis, often in childhood, without being aware of it. His or her T-lymphocytes have evidently swarmed to the lesion, overcome the invading bacteria, and sealed off the pocket of infection with a scar in the lung. (Radiologists quite frequently sound a lung cancer alarm only to find that the ominous opacities visualized in the chest by x-rays are remnant scars of a case of tuberculosis that may have produced only a transient fever and a minor cough at the time, perhaps years or decades before.) At any rate, once the antigen, in this case some substance belonging to the TB bacillus, has been recognized and attacked by the competent immune cells of a human or animal, the system is cocked for a much more rapid and massive attack the next time around. Thus a tiny infusion of tuberculin antigen into the skin will not produce any reaction in a person who has never harbored the germ. But the identical quantity of tuberculin antigen will cause an angry sore in anyone who has ever had or who currently has tuberculosis. A massively amplified immune reaction has been triggered. Millions of lymphocytes answer the challenge within hours, rushing to respond to an alarm that may not have been sounded for many years. Hence the term "delayed hypersensitivity."

Similarly, an animal that has received a graft of skin from another not its twin (and "twin" in this context denotes an individual derived from generations of inbreeding such that sibling mice or rats after half a dozen generations of mating brothers and sisters with each other have virtually identical sets of genes) will reject much more rapidly a second graft from the same incompatible animal.

Like any society composed of disparate elements, the body must have systems to enforce order. The white blood cells, generally termed leukocytes, appear to be the major elements of this police system, whether they are circulating in the bloodstream or manning outposts in the lymph nodes whence they can survey the fluid lymph that bathes all cells (except those in the brain and spinal cord) as it returns from the tissues into the venous blood.* The system is established at a very early age, but evidently not so early that it cannot be circumvented. In an earlier chapter of this book, I mentioned the classic example of tolerance induction in mice by Medawar and his colleagues in London in the 1950s. A second method was also uncovered in London, in 1961 by Dr. J. F. A. P. Miller of the Chester Beatty Research Institute. A few years earlier, there had been published evidence that the thymus gland had some regulatory influence over the number of lymphocytes in circulation, thus offering a hint that the mysterious gland might play a role in leukemia. (Leukemia is a form of cancer in which immature white blood cells take over the bloodstream, causing disruptions to vital body function comparable to what might occur if every, say, eight-year-old child in a major city suddenly gained the capability of turning into two children every forty-eight hours. For each original child there would be almost 20,000 offspring in the first month alone and their hordes might be expected to battle the rest of the population for the available sustenance.)

Miller, seeking to learn more about the thymus because of its possible role in leukemia, decided to cut the pinhead-sized glands out of newborn mice to see what sort of disability they might suffer. It was well known by this time that removal of the thymus from an adult animal produced no disastrous effects. But Miller found that newborn mice lacking the tiny gland died in a couple of months, their lymph nodes and spleens in a state of shrunken uselessness. Miller tried grafting skin from unrelated mice. The grafts survived. He tried rat skin, even more markedly foreign. The grafts from rats took, too. Since it was not

* For a detailed discussion of the various types of leukocytes and their specialized functions and developments, see Roger Lewin, *In Defense of the Body: An Introduction to the New Immunology* (New York: Anchor Press/Doubleday, 1974).

then possible to isolate any hormone or other substance secreted by the thymus gland, it seemed that lymphocytes in charge of the delayed hypersensitivity reaction needed the gland in order to perform their function of protecting the body against strangers. Later, by the use of thymus transplantation under very special conditions, it was learned that some lymphocytes need to live in the thymus for a while to gain the ability to specialize in defense later on and that the gland secretes some substance that endows these lymphocytes with their mature function when they leave the thymus and circulate.

Good, in Minnesota, had by searching back through evolution for animals that had only rudimentary recognition of strangeness found that such tolerant creatures lacked a thymus. During the period when Miller was thymectomizing his mice in London, Good had suggested to two of his juniors at Minnesota that they remove the thymus from rabbits. The results at Minnesota, too, were suggestive of a close relationship between cellular immunity and the thymus. But Good's trainee doctors had not found it feasible to take the gland from the baby rabbits until they were five days old. In that brief period, the newborn animals were able, with the aid of their thymus glands, to set up at least some of the white-cell immune system. Though the results, therefore, were more ambiguous than those of Miller, Good was able to draw similar conclusions.

The next experiments were aimed at finding out why thymectomized mice died so young. Techniques had been developed, notably at Notre Dame University, for delivering infant animals by Caesarian section and into a totally sterile, germ-free environment. Animals thymectomized, but thus protected from bacteria and viruses, thrived. Scientists drew the obvious conclusion. The role of the thymus was to initiate part of the immunologic protective mechanism and especially to put into action the cellular, as opposed to the antibody—or humoral—sector.

Until 1943 little attention had been given to tumors as antigens. Since cancer arose in the body of the host or victim, it seemed unlikely that cancer cells would bear any markers identifiable by the patient as strange or foreign. Yet, of course, there were hundreds of cases where, indisputably, a patient with cancer had in some unaided fashion dissolved the tumor and cured himself. Working at the Bronx Veterans Administration Hospital Ludwik Gross provided an answer that was not confirmed in more sophisticated and exacting tests and therefore not accepted for a decade. Gross used colonies of inbred mice. He first showed, as was to be expected, that tumors induced in the mice by a coal tar derivative, methylcholanthrene, would be readily accepted by a twin and would grow and kill the animal. But Gross speculated that if a genetic change was involved in tumor formation, whether the change was produced by a chemical, a virus, or radiation, there should be one or more different proteins made by the unruly cells. If this were true, then a genetic duplicate of the mouse with the tumor should still be able to recognize and reject its littermate's cancer under appropriate circumstances. The delayed hypersensitivity reaction was one possibility. So Dr. Gross put tumors into twins and a few days later surgically removed them before they could kill the recipients. He had now, possibly, cocked the cellular immune weapon. When a comparable slice of tumor taken from a twin was sewn into a recipient mouse for the second time, a few weeks after surgical removal of the first tumor implant, the animal destroyed it successfully without outside assistance and survived.

There were, evidently, specific tumor antigens as well as tissue, species and individual (transplantation) markers. Why, then, did not the body's defenses recognize and reject tumor cells as quickly and as effectively as they did grafts of mismatched skin, blood, and other transplants? Two decades later this riddle is still being studied intensively. That is why the arrival of Dr. Summerlin and his mouse-skin grafting at a cancer center was not so far removed from tumor research as might at first be supposed. There was the hope that Summerlin's work, with its promise of casting new light on tolerance and rejection of tissues, might also tell science something about the enigma of cancer.

6
STAG AND HOUNDS

THE YEAR 1974 should have been one of gratification for Lewis Thomas, the sixty-year-old physician elevated to the presidency of the Memorial Sloan-Kettering Cancer Center a year before. His slender volume of biological essays, *The Lives of a Cell*, was about to be published, and he was beginning to understand, if not control, the power structures of Memorial Hospital and its sister research institute. Later, in the spring, his book would climb to the New York *Times* best-seller list and, in

1975, win the National Book Award. Yet all this was of little comfort to him when the Summerlin incident exploded.

When he was asked later whether he didn't, on that cruel March day, feel a little as former President Nixon must have on a day in June of 1972 when he first heard of the Watergate burglary, Thomas replied with his usual care that he did not. "It was, obviously, a very difficult problem. It was difficult for Dr. Good and Dr. Old and all the senior members of the institute. It was also difficult for me, but it was not really a terribly complicated problem in the sense that there were arrays of choices and options among various courses of action. It seemed to me then, as it seems to me now in retrospect, that there was only one thing to do. The man involved was suspended and a committee of his peers representing the scientific community was appointed to look into the affair."

Yet it is odd that the head of an institution dependent upon public support, the government, and conservative businessmen to whom scandal would be anathema, did not consult the center's lawyers at the earliest moment.

No written word about the trouble circulated within or outside the institution, though its public relations director had a brief statement he was authorized to give the press in case there was a leak. It was only on May 3, two weeks after the leak had sprung, that Good formalized the appointment of a committee of his Sloan-Kettering peers to investigate the Summerlin claims with a letter to the committee chairman and a Sloan-Kettering vice-president, C. Chester Stock.

Later, Thomas was to say, "The . . . letter was written with my approval and concurrence, and confirmed verbal action which had been taken by Dr. Good, pursuant to which the Peer Review Committee commenced investigation on April 5, 1974."

There was no way to contain the sordid story. The larger scientific community was painfully aware both of the reported breakthrough in postculture transplantation and of Good's endorsement of the young skin specialist as a scientist worthy of attention. Only a few weeks before the inking of the mice there had been a nasty scene when another eminent immunologist had learned he was to share the podium at the Rockefeller University seminar with Summerlin.

What would the press write of this fraud at one of the nation's most prestigious cancer centers? What would the scientific community say in letters to editors? What would be the reaction of the National Cancer Institute, which was now reconsidering a grant to Summerlin? How would the donating public react to what the press might report? Last but not least, how would Summerlin himself respond to the humiliation, word of which was spreading fast among his peers?

In short, the Summerlin episode could not have erupted at a worse time for an institution whose senior scientists were openly displaying insubordination and telling all who would listen, off the record, of their discontent. It could not have come at a more crucial time financially. In addition, it would, when it became public knowledge, fuel the suspicions surrounding science and scientists.

With the collaboration of Drs. Good and Old, Dr. Thomas approved the review committee. Its chairman, Dr. Stock, had been serving until Dr. Good's arrival as deputy to Sloan-Kettering's retiring director, Dr. Wade. Stock was as nonpartisan a figure as the center could muster. A man who speaks carefully and thinks before he utters a word, the sixty-four-year-old biochemist was a natural choice. To work with him, he had Dr. Burchenal, also a charter Sloan-Kettering member, and a co-winner of a Lasker award for his work on the chemotherapy of leukemia. Burchenal, Princeton-educated with an M.D. from Johns Hopkins is in some ways Stock's opposite, impatient, a rapid talker, very much at home in any situation. Like Stock, Joe Burchenal is totally devoted to the institute and its goals on every level. Old and Good named another expert in leukemia, but from a more theoretical, experimental standpoint, Dr. Bayard D. Clarkson, like Burchenal a Princeton graduate, who had been a member of the institute since 1958. Clarkson is a big, ruddy-faced man in his late forties whose basic shyness conceals an extraordinary grasp of the most recondite aspects of cell replication, a matter vital to the understanding of cancer.

Dr. Martin Sonenberg, the fourth committee member, is as familiar with hormonal action as Clarkson is with cellular dynamics. Both an M.D. and a Ph.D., he has been with Sloan-Kettering since 1949. The fifth member of the committee was Dr. Boyse, a

diminutive, generously maned Englishman and a close associate
of Dr. Old in pioneering immunologic research involving the antigens of cells that enable them to identify each other. Boyse,
who had been a member of the institute since 1961, is known for
his sweet disposition and had remained aloof from the feuding
over Good's changes at the institute. Finally, in a bow to Summerlin's most recent habitat in Minneapolis, Good named to the
committee Dr. John W. Hadden, appointed an associate member
of the institute on his arrival from the University of Minnesota,
who was a clinical immunologist. Summerlin was evidently unhappy with the choice of the Minnesota researcher, and midway
in the investigation he made known his objections to Stock.
Rather than add still another controversial element to an already
sticky situation, Hadden resigned, leaving five members to judge
Summerlin's scientific work and his behavior. Although all of the
five were long-term members of the institute, none of them belonged to the rebellious junta that had brought their gripes
about Good's authoritarian stance to the attention of Thomas.

It was clear to everyone that both mentor and protégé were in
the dock. The jury of five would be fair. No question about that.
There was little doubt in anyone's mind that it would find
Summerlin guilty of at least one transgression of the code of
science: Thou shalt not fake thy data. What was less clear was
what attitude the peer review committee would adopt with respect to their boss, Dr. Good.

While the investigation committee was being appointed,
science reporters in New York and Washington were garnering
tales of dissension at the cancer center. A remark here, a snide
comment there revealed that Good's first year at Sloan-Kettering had not gone smoothly for all concerned. The tales of
infighting between the old guard and the new weren't solid
enough to produce "hard" news or a feature article, but they
served to focus the writers' collective attention on Sixty-eighth
Street as they awaited developments.

One who watched as closely as anybody was Barbara Yuncker,
medical reporter for the tabloid New York *Post*. She had been
raised in Indiana reading newspapers where the first rule for reporters is to mind your own territory and the rest of the nation

will take care of itself. Except for weekend forays to her country house about 110 miles north of New York City, Yuncker keeps a very close watch on the medical happenings of New York from her brownstone in the West Twenties, and she keeps readers of the *Post* well informed about medicine and medical politics in Manhattan and its neighboring boroughs. There are few skeletons in the well-stocked closets of New York's medical establishment that have escaped the eye of this experienced reporter, winner of two Lasker awards for medical journalism.

How the *Post's* writer heard about Summerlin's inked mice remains her secret. However, in making her telephonic rounds of her beat, she learned of the episode—but not the name of the perpetrator—on Wednesday, April 10, confirmed it, found out that the painter was Good's young associate, and put in a call to Thomas on Friday when she had her facts pretty well buttoned down.

Yuncker had written earlier in the *Post* of Summerlin's transplants after organ culture on the say-so of Good. Most reporters have a strong tendency to identify themselves with the articles they write, though it is a rare reader who can remember the byline atop any given story. A later implication that the story might have had a flimsy basis is taken by the writer as a personal affront. He or she worries about lack of perception, about not, perhaps, asking shrewd enough questions, about not checking with enough outside sources, and so forth.

So it can be assumed that Yuncker's conversations with Thomas and Good over the Easter-Passover weekend of 1974 were not devoid of asperity. All I know is that she spoke briefly with Thomas and at considerable length with Good the next day.

It was not that Thomas hadn't been expecting the call; he just didn't know from whom it would come. He had no handy denial that he could live with later on. He had only the barebones statement, composed with the aid of his public affairs director, confirming that Summerlin had been suspended pending an investigation by fellow scientists. Yuncker broke the story on Monday afternoon, April 15.

But if this seemed to ease the tension for Thomas and his subordinates, there was worse to come at the hands of the

Times's Jane Brody. It could not have been a pleasure for her to read in the pages of a rival newspaper that one of her articles, the one written in some haste at Nogales the year before, concerned achievements by a doctor who faked experimental results, or was at least alleged to have done so.

The New York *Times* has the largest staff of science reporters of any newspaper in the nation, almost twice as many, indeed, as the Associated Press. Few of them are to be found in the home office on any given day or even in the home city. Since the newspaper considers itself a national publication, there are many scientific and medical meetings, expeditions, and other technical stories to be covered all over the country. The *Times* does not stint on such coverage. As a result, however, the paper's own backyard is not well raked.

When, for example, Sloan-Kettering had copies of a press release announcing Good's appointment hand-delivered to the city desk and the science department of the *Times* for publication the following day, not a word of the appointment appeared in the following day's paper. Returning to her office from a trip that Friday, Brody groaned when told of her paper's delinquency and set the matter to rights with an article on Saturday. Now, however, in April 1974, what she had to set to rights was the warranty that Good appeared to have erroneously issued for Summerlin. She did this by opening up for public inspection the dissension and the gripes that some institute staffers had been airing since Good's arrival.

The *Times* story, which appeared April 17, 1974, began, "An allegation that a young physician-scientist at the Memorial Sloan-Kettering Cancer Center here falsified potentially important research findings has caused widespread dismay among scientists both in and out of the famed institution.

"In interviews with the New York *Times* yesterday, the scientists, most of whom asked not to be quoted by name, said that the episode reflected dangerous trends in current efforts to gain scientific acclaim and funds for research, as well as possible misdirection of research at Sloan-Kettering itself." After noting that Dr. Summerlin declined comment on the affair, Brody continued: "Among the criticisms that have been leveled are the fol-

lowing: That Dr. Good . . . had publicized too highly Dr. Summerlin's early results—possibly for publicity purposes—even
though no one else had been able to reproduce them . . . That
Dr. Good failed to supervise Dr. Summerlin's work closely
enough . . . That Dr. Good has staffed the institution with a
large group of young, unproven scientists whom he has placed
under great pressure to produce results . . . That, according to
one of Dr. Good's long-time admirers, instead of building on the
work of established investigators at Sloan-Kettering, Dr. Good
has chosen 'to shoot for the spectacular' and in the process has
'manipulated national attention and attracted an enormous
amount of money for the Institute.'"

The *Times* reporter needed something in her article, which
followed the *Post*'s by two days, that would give it greater depth
and comprehensiveness, qualities the *Times* holds very dear. She
had found it, but it was bitter gall for the staff of the cancer
center, or, at least, for those of them not numbered among the
dissidents. It may be conjectured that it was the first *Times* article that suggested to Summerlin that he was not entirely lacking
in ammunition if he cared to fight back.

Still worse was coming for Sloan-Kettering in the pages of
Science. Another writer endowed with a formidable reportorial
intelligence and a willingness to use it in skewering the powerful
was marshaling her contacts. Barbara Culliton's article ran on
parts of six pages in the May 10, 1974, issue of the most widely
read U.S. general scientific journal and the weekly organ of the
American Association for the Advancement of Science. Titled
"The Sloan-Kettering Affair: A Story Without a Hero," Culliton's
piece read in part: "Beyond the alleged mouse painting incident
is the question now on many persons' minds of the validity of the
whole of Summerlin's work during the last four years, work
which potentially has enormous implications for research in immunology and cancer.

"Second, there is the reputation of Good, Summerlin's boss and
mentor, a tremendously powerful and persuasive man who has
lent the prestige of his own stature to the work Summerlin has
been doing.

"Third, there is the reputation and internal stability of Sloan-

Kettering itself, a troubled institution that has been struggling for the last couple of years to find its identity and its future.

"The present crisis could turn out to be ruinous for all three."

Culliton also drew a conclusion that Summerlin was later to echo in his defense. Her piece ended: "Sloan-Kettering these days is not a happy place. It is rich and getting richer, but not happy. In 1972, the research institute and its affiliate, Memorial Hospital, received about $7 million in government grants and contracts. According to the National Cancer Institute, the Memorial Sloan-Kettering Cancer Center will get about $20 million in fiscal 1975, more than any other cancer center in the country. For that amount of money, people are going to expect to see results, whether in clinical or basic research. If the present crisis generated by the Summerlin case is any indication, it appears that a high-pressure environment that drives individuals to exaggeration and fosters hostility is not ideal for the kind of achievements in research that Good, like everyone else, would like to see . . ."

The major news weeklies also hinted at the same theme in their initial coverage of the story. All of the writers involved were obviously aware of the misgivings voiced in many quarters by many scientists and research administrators about the wisdom of going all out against cancer with a big escalation in funding before anyone really knew whether cancer was, in fact, one disease or a dozen in terms either of causation or optimal therapy. The Summerlin-Good debacle appeared to bear out the point that Culliton emphasized, even though her figure on 1975 support for Memorial Sloan-Kettering looks to have been somewhat inflated by her source at the NCI.

How high emotion was running at the institute may be gauged from an episode that had occurred in Atlantic City only a few days after the *Times* article ran and before the *Science* piece appeared. The huge annual meeting of the Federation of American Societies for Experimental Biology was in progress, and a panel discussion of the relationship between scientists and the press had been scheduled. A member of the panel was Lawrence K. Altman, M.D., medical reporter for the New York *Times,* and probably the only medical doctor to be so employed by any U.S.

newspaper. Altman usually does not run about reporting hard news of breaking medical stories, preferring instead to write roundup articles in which a variety of approaches to and opinions of a medical problem can be presented.

The problem of the News coverage accorded Summerlin's transplants seemed to Altman to be worth raising as an example of the state of affairs that ensues when widespread confirmation of new findings has been preceded by a blast of press, television, and radio reports hailing a breakthrough. He inserted his comments into his prepared text at the last moment, believing the problem to be both timely and apropos for mention at the Federation session.

When, following Altman's presentation, discussion was permitted from the attending biologists and physicians, a professor of medicine at the University of California, San Francisco, and a widely respected researcher in the field of immunology, took the microphone to say that the Summerlin affair was a perfect example of why careful scientists were so wary of talking to the press until their work had been properly published. Altman said he thought that most of Summerlin's work had appeared in one journal or another. This was not a strong enough defense for Joanne Good. Mrs. Good, who obviously felt that her husband was being criticized by innuendo, insisted that all of Summerlin's work had been properly reviewed and published. The panel's moderator curtly cut her off, explaining that the session was not going to be devoted to a wrangle over the Summerlin scandal.

During the first week after his suspension Summerlin, probably on the advice of his lawyers, was maintaining a discreet silence at home in Darien. When *Medical World News* reached him for comment, he said he hoped he would be invited to appear before the peer review committee but that he did not then know its membership and had not yet been invited to present his case. He eventually made his appearance before Dr. Stock's committee on May 10.

Had Summerlin attended an early April meeting of the American Burn Association, he would have received another shock. He was scheduled to present the final paper of the meeting but pleaded illness. It was just as well. Surgeons from burn centers in Cincinnati, Miami, and Dallas were going to respond to the Sloan-Kettering researcher's claims of further successes in human skin grafting by reporting their failures. Dr. Bruce Mac-Millan told *Medical World News* that even when attempts were made to culture and then graft skin from a closely matched donor, the grafts all failed within ninety days, lasting only slightly longer than freshly excised skin. Dr. MacMillan, president of the burn association and head of dermatologic research at the Cincinnati Shriners Burns Institute, said his group was astonished, since they used Summerlin's techniques, when the grafts were sloughed off. They, too, had sent a delegation to the Sloan-Kettering Institute to find out what they had been doing wrong. The news of the painted mice produced a considerable sense of relief in many transplantation research laboratories around the country, where guilt feelings over failure to reproduce the Summerlin results had been the paramount emotion.

But the other shoe had not yet been dropped. All during the first weeks of May Dr. Stock's committee was plowing through papers, checking back at Minnesota, telephoning immunologists around the country, and, of course, interviewing Drs. Good, Raaf, Ninnemann, and the others directly involved at Sloan-Kettering and also Drs. Laino and Mondino from across York Avenue at Cornell.

Friday, May 24, presented New Yorkers with a rare gift, a warm and sunny spring morning. Reporters arriving at 9 A.M. at the wide entrance to the new Memorial Hospital building could hear birds chirping in the trees surrounding Rockefeller University across the avenue. Inside the long, carefully guarded hospital conference room, however, solemnity reigned. There were no TV cameras and no microphones except those attached to small personal tape recorders. The score of journalists present had been carefully screened for the first unveiling of the twenty-two page peer review committee's report. They were ushered into the room, offered coffee and a bun, and given the report plus a seven-page statement that Thomas was to read as an introduction. Summerlin was not present, but one of his female colleagues and a supporter was—or tried to be.

She was Dr. E. R. Lappano-Coletta, who occupied an office adjacent to that of the suspended scientist over in the Kettering Laboratory. She trudged down the hospital corridor, a short, stocky, and evidently perturbed figure, and she made a fuss when the guard at the door told her she couldn't come in. When reporters asked why she had been excluded, Good responded that she had recently been informed that her appointment as a researcher at Sloan-Kettering had not been renewed and that, in consequence, she had been upset and given to bursting in on meetings and shouting at people.

Aside from this interlude, the press conference was a scene of utter decorum. The three female writers who had caused the cancer center officials so much consternation were reading their committee reports as were a half-dozen medical and news weekly magazine reporters and those from the Washington *Post*, the New York *Daily News*, and the two wire services, Associated Press and United Press International. Thomas, Stock, and Good sat at the head of the table, the latter wearing a snowy white coat over his customary turtleneck sweater so that a heavy silver emblem hanging by a black cord around his neck was barely visible. Thomas and Stock wore business suits, no lab coats. Good doodled on a pad as Thomas read his statement.

Thomas read from a letter sent to Stock by Good on May 3 officially confirming the appointment of the six-man committee. Reviewing briefly the misrepresentation of the corneal transplants in the rabbits and the admitted doctoring of the mice, Thomas announced that the trustees of the center had decided, based on the committee's report handed to them four days previously, to terminate Summerlin's relationship with the hospital and institute.

The Memorial Sloan-Kettering head then offered his own explanation of what had been going on: ". . . after discussion with Dr. Summerlin, his wife, and his personal psychiatrist, I have concluded that the most rational explanation for Dr. Summerlin's recent performance is that he has been suffering from an emotional disturbance of such a nature that he has not been fully responsible for the actions he has taken or the representations he has made. Accordingly, it has been agreed that the Center will

provide Dr. Summerlin with a period of medical leave on full
salary ($40,000) beginning now, for up to one year to enable
him to obtain the rest and professional care that his condition
may require." (The immediate cost to the institute was far
higher, however. Stock estimated that the committee had met
seven times over a three-week period and that its six original
members had each spent no fewer than 150 hours on the investigation.)

Now Thomas turned his attention to the man in the turtleneck sitting to his left. He read from his statement slowly in his
somewhat raspy voice: "'The peer review committee report includes the following. "Thorough inquiry supports the conclusion
that Dr. Good did not knowingly misrepresent any of the facts
connected with the Summerlin work. Any misconceptions that
Dr. Good may have held were essentially acquired from Dr.
Summerlin.

"'It would appear that the great demands made on Dr. Good,
especially after he took over the directorship, compromised his
ability to personally supervise projects of Dr. Summerlin that
conspicuously lacked the sound experimental planning and guidance that Dr. Good could have provided in other circumstances.'"

Dr. Thomas continued: "'It is evident from the peer review
committee's report that Dr. Good began to have personal misgivings about the validity of Dr. Summerlin's work sometime
around mid-November 1973. At that time, Dr. Good assigned responsibility to two other scientists within SKI to attempt dupli-
cation of the reported skin graft work . . . During this same
period it is now apparent that certain scientists within SKI also
had serious misgivings regarding the reportedly successful corneal transplants, although there is no evidence that Dr. Good
was clearly aware of these doubts.

"'Dr. Good has expressed to the board of trustees his feeling,
in retrospect, that he should have been quicker to perceive and
uncover the deficiencies in Dr. Summerlin's scientific data. However, the board of trustees is of the opinion that the time-consuming nature of the tremendous responsibilities carried by Dr.
Good in the period following his appointment to the direc-

torship of SKI in January 1973 placed him in an extremely difficult situation, and it is understandable, and indeed inevitable, that during this time it may have been impossible for him to maintain the close, day-to-day supervision which, viewed now in retrospect, might have prevented or terminated more quickly this regrettable affair.'"

The report of the committee went into painstaking and painful detail about Summerlin's misrepresentations of the corneal transplants both to *Medical World News* in March that year and to another physicians' publication, *Clinical Trends in Ophthalmology, Laryngology and Allergy,* in April. In both instances writers and editors for the publications had carefully checked caption material for a rabbit's eye photograph supplied by Summerlin with him. One of the reporters, Jean Watson, Ph.D., had, the committee report noted, forwarded to Summerlin the account of his successful corneal cultures for him to read and correct. Based on her records, Watson supplied evidence that even after the mouse caper and his suspension from the Institute on March 26 Summerlin continued to play out his hand. She received the cleared copy from Summerlin on April 1, six days after the fateful early-morning visit to Good's office.

Good, recalling later how completely he had been hoodwinked over the corneal transplants, could even muster a chuckle remembering the episode. He related, "It was in late September of 1973, I think, that Summerlin first showed me these rabbits, and he showed me the rejecting cornea on the one hand and the clear one in the other eye and he said, 'Now this is the cultured cornea,' and I said, 'My God! That is the most fantastic thing I ever saw in my life.' And then I said, 'But you know, Bill, the thing is I can't even see that that eye has been operated on.' And he says, 'Oh, these men over at Cornell are master surgeons, and they're doing limbus-to-limbus total corneal transplants. And I said, 'Limbus to limbus! That's more than you can expect, that's fantastic.' So I showed the rabbits to several people later on. There were ten of them over in the animal quarters in Kettering. He had shown me how they did the surgery with pictures of one eye with the sutures in place. Of course, I know now that those were early photographs of unsuccessful operations before rejection had set in. But they were beautiful transplants and it just didn't seem conceivable that there was no rejection whatsoever. Whenever he presented that at staff meetings and so on, it was presented as this new method of corneal transplantation. "Well, we had done work at Minnesota. Dr. Miller from the ophthalmology department had come over to work with Dr. Summerlin and he had done some corneal transplants with small pieces of cultured tissue in the middle of the rabbit's eye and there was no question that survival of the graft was prolonged. Whether those data will hold up remains to be seen. Dr. Doughman is working on that."

(Dr. Donald Doughman—pronounced "Doofman"—is a Boston ophthalmologist who undertook verification of the Minnesota corneal work late in 1972. He has said, "Our initial findings were just glorious. We really thought we had something. We didn't graft human [cadaver] corneas, but we outbred and cross-bred our rabbits to make them as incompatible as possible genetically. The results at Minnesota were intriguing, and there was no question of falsifying—you can't paint a cornea on an eye. But as soon as I learned about Bill Summerlin's problems, it was obvious to me I had been assuming it had to work because he made it work on skin." But the combination of Summerlin's enthusiasm and Good's backing it set Dr. Doughman back by at least a year. He told reporter Lois Wingerson of *Medical World News* that after doing five hundred rabbits he was going to begin his study all over again because of his suspicions of wishful thinking. More money down the drain.)

The peer review committee, though, had still another catastrophe to report. It concerned the "Old Man," the only long-term survivor from Summerlin's Minnesota days still bearing grafted skin. Said the committee's report, "It is not in dispute that in Dr. Summerlin's [animal] quarters the only mouse carrying a fully accepted skin allograft which had been retained over a long period, since Dr. Summerlin's arrival at M[emorial] S[loan-] K[ettering] C[ancer] C[enter] . . . was one nicknamed 'The Old Man' . . . After the blackening episode, Dr. Good asked Dr. Boyse to test this mouse to decide whether it might be an F_1 hybrid, which could explain the acceptance of white (albino) skin by an agouti (wild-type speckled coat) recipient solely on a well-known genetic basis. By inspection alone, a C3H mouse cannot be distinguished from a hybrid between the C3H and A mouse strains.

". . . The 'Old Man' had been grafted on 11/22/1971, according to the label on the cage. Tests in the laboratory of Dr. Boyse, carried out on blood taken from this mouse on 4/3/74, reveal it to be a hybrid. . . .

"The committee found it difficult to credit that Dr. Summerlin could have been continuously ignorant of this elementary possibility, which became ever more critical as this mouse assumed the role of a single exceptional success, or that he remained unaware that simple tests by any of several colleagues could immediately have settled the matter."

On top of this studied naïvete of Summerlin, the committee cited contradictory statements that Summerlin had made in grant applications in 1973 for which they could find no properly tabulated mouse data.

Finally, thoroughly puzzled by almost complete lack of coherent data and of surviving, successfully grafted mice, the committee asked Summerlin what had happened to all the other animals he was claiming as successes: "Dr. Summerlin gave the astonishing reply that they were sacrificed at intervals to provide serum to be stored for H-2 [histocompatibility] antibody tests at a later date. It is scarcely conceivable that Dr. Summerlin could have believed, in such immunologically sophisticated surroundings as Dr. Good's group at Minnesota, that it is necessary to kill a mouse to obtain serum." The report demolished Summerlin's defenses one by one. (See Appendix 1 at the end of this book for the full report.)

If Thomas and the Memorial Sloan-Kettering trustees were content to accept Good's busyness as an excuse for backing Summerlin and putting his name on his protégé's research papers, some members of the press were not. (Good had at least insisted on Summerlin revising a paper he was about to submit to the *Journal of Experimental Medicine* in November of 1973. The tables of mouse successes and failures didn't accurately represent the numbers of animals cited in the accompanying text. Good

warned his associate that he didn't want to be embarrassed by
having the report rejected by the editors as too sloppy for
publication. This rebuke came at precisely the time when Summerlin's close associates started noticing the change in his previously cheerful demeanor.)

But the questioning at the Memorial Hospital press conference
was at first subdued. How much of Summerlin's work, then,
was invalid? Thomas answered, "I retain an open mind and I
believe longer graft survival has been demonstrated after cells
are cultured." Nobody pressed Thomas to define how much
longer was "longer" in his view. The head of the center added
that growing corneal cells in culture appeared to offer some advantages in storage by allowing eye surgeons more time in which
to try to match up donors and recipients.

Then Good joined in. "Dr. Summerlin came to our group
in the fall of 1971 with five years' work in this area. He worked
on from one to two thousand mice while at Minnesota." Good
went on to echo Thomas' hunch that there was some validity in
the skin culturing research and some benefit to be derived by
culturing corneas.

Brushing aside these faint attempts at optimism, the *Times*'s
Jane Brody went to the issue that was gnawing the assembled
writers but which was left unmentioned in the committee's report. Why had Good continued to enthuse to the press and
others about the Summerlin findings long after his November
1973 misgivings? You could see the immunologist stiffen, but his
slightly adenoidal baritone was muted as he replied. "Jane, I
always said *if* the work can be repeated. I said that *if* it was
repeated, it was of the greatest importance."

Stuart Auerbach of the Washington *Post* jumped in: "Didn't
you ever notice that Summerlin's lab was a shambles according
to this report?"

Good reverted to his earlier reply, amplifying it a little: "Dr.
Summerlin came as a scientist who had achieved acclaim as a
scientist. I outlined a program for him of analyzing mouse-skin
transplantations crossing major tissue-compatibility barriers and
specified which strains he was to use." Warming to his subject
and denying that Summerlin's area was a shambles, Good

seemed to enjoy relating how a prominent cancer immunologist, Dr. Donald Morton of the University of California, had picked up one of Summerlin's mice and shaken it hard by its tuft of guinea-pig hair but had failed to dislodge the graft. But then he added that the graft had been sloughed off at "three to four months."

It was getting harder and harder for the writers to make out whether the scientist was or was not still standing by his protégé, still believing the few shreds left of his work, because he wanted to believe so badly. Whether Summerlin's year at the center had been worth a budget for his lab and clinical work of over $200,000 hung in the air.

Seeming to waver in his attitude, Good related how Ninnemann had warned him the corneal claims were false, but he said, "I didn't believe him until March when I spoke to Dr. Laino and he told me it was complete crud."

Jane Brody was still not satisfied. "Did you ever check with the Stanford investigators or examine the patients' grafts?" (She has since said that she checked with Karasek and that he told her he considered the Summerlin grafts only a slightly superior form of wound dressing.) Good answered that he had himself examined only slides of tissue taken from two of the successful human grafts. One, from a black man grafted with a white person's skin had not impressed him, Good said, because healing skin can lose its pigmentation. The other, from a male patient grafted with female skin, had shown Barr bodies four years after the surgery. That had impressed him, the scientist said, because if the skin had been the man's own, it should not have exhibited Barr bodies, the shriveled remnant of the woman's extra X chromosome. (Men, having for sex chromosomes both an X and a Y as opposed to the female's double X should, theoretically, not have Barr bodies, but some of their cells seem to.)

Later Good explained to me that though a minority of male skin cells may show what looks like a Barr body and though as many as 40 per cent of cells in female skin may not show the chromosomal remnant, the skin of the female donor in question was especially rich in Barr bodies and therefore he felt the identification was adequate. The trouble is that how the cells are

sliced and stained makes a great difference in determining the
presence or absence of Barr bodies, and Good had never gotten
from Summerlin details of the technique employed.

At least one of the scientists now working for Good at the institute disagrees with him. Dr. Bijan Safai, came to Memorial
Sloan-Kettering from New York University Medical Center's
well-known Skin and Cancer Clinic in July of 1973 to work with
Dr. Summerlin. Dr. Safai, who is the only other physician at Memorial to have performed a graft with human skin taken from
one of Dr. Summerlin's cultures, says flatly that Barr-body count-
ing to determine survival of a female skin graft on a male or vice
versa is hopelessly inaccurate and invalid.

On the other hand, Safai performed his graft on March 28,
1974, two days after Summerlin's departure, and as of July of
that year it seemed to him to be working well. The patient, a
skid-row bum, had been sent up from Bellevue Hospital. At
Bellevue, the man's frost-bitten foot had been about to be ampu-
tated because of an unhealing ulcer. Safai told me that the
graft of cells from Summerlin's skin bank seemed to take well
and had evidently saved the foot. Though he had biopsied
(sampled) the graft seven times by July, Safai could draw
no hard-and-fast conclusions about what was happening and
whether the graft really took.

The committee had looked into the rosy reports of successful
grafts made by Summerlin during his stay at Sloan-Kettering. Its report observed that Stanford's Karasek supported
Summerlin's claims of prolonged survival when he rose to
comment on a presentation by the dermatologist at the May 1973
meeting of the American Society for Clinical Investigation.

Once at Memorial Hospital, the report continued, Summerlin had operated on four patients, applying cultured cells
from his skin bank. One, an alcoholic, had a big ulcer as a result
of an accident; one had psoriasis and had developed an ulcer as
a result of X-ray treatment of his disfiguring skin disease; the
third patient suffered ulceration as a result of impaired blood
circulation; and the fourth had a similar problem related to
poorly controlled diabetes.

In three of these cases, the committee believed there was good evidence that the grafts of cultured cells had survived longer than would grafts of freshly excised skin from an incompatible donor. In the fourth patient, the graft had become infected and was lost quite early. Including Safai's patient, the committee concluded, "Thus in four of these five patients there appeared to be an increase in the time during which the graft persisted despite an underlying impairment of [blood] circulation which militated against graft survival. In the two persisting grafts the possibility of a permanent take had not been ruled out. "One of the two is Dr. Safai's patient, while the other was the alcoholic, who left the hospital with his graft in place three weeks after the surgery but had not returned or been found.

There seemed, then, to be some grounds for Good's defense of therapy with cultured skin but not enough to argue a breach of the Burnet-Medawar dogma.

The journalists' questioning at the May 24 conference then turned to broader issues. Was the Summerlin episode, as had been suggested in several articles, an example of too much pressure and temptation for a young physician-researcher? The three cancer center officials indicated that none of them felt that to be the case. Thomas said, "In thirty-five years this is the first misrepresentation I've encountered," and he added after a pause, "I can't accept this as fraud, pure and simple." Several writers present who were working or had worked on articles for newspaper city editors thought silently about what their bosses would have said had they been caught fabricating an interview or throwing into their stories a few colorful but imagined items. Fraud, in such a case, would likely be the kindest epithet applied to them and two weeks' pay their maximum stake while they tried to find another job.

Good's reply to a question about why he had installed Summerlin as a full member of the institute has been dealt with in Chapter 2. He said at the press conference, "I'm not sure why Dr. Summerlin wasn't reviewed by the vice-presidents." The simplest answer was clearly that the vice-presidents of the Sloan-Kettering Institute probably would not have accepted so untried a scientist even as an associate member. But Good promised that future appointees would be reviewed by a new Council of Field Coordinators and that the Sloan-Kettering senate would have more of a voice "in a few more months."

Jane Brody asked how Summerlin could have told her at the Nogales luncheon that cultured and transplanted adrenal glands had kept mice alive for eight months whereas other animals with freshly grafted adrenal glands had quickly died. (The committee had evaluated Summerlin's claims in this area as statistically untenable.) Good avoided a direct answer to this question, saying only, "My promulgation of Dr. Summerlin's work was based on a major dermatology prize [that of the Pacific Dermatological Association in 1972] and his scientific publications; and my enthusiasm gave him more prominence than he would otherwise have had."

These concluding remarks left hanging the very question the writers had come to the cancer hospital that sunny May morning to pursue. But another distraction was already in preparation. It came, of course, from the man Thomas might justifiably have figured was all buttoned up in penitence with the $40,000. Since the Monday following the Memorial Hospital press conference was, aptly enough, Memorial Day, Summerlin invited the press to his suburban Connecticut house on Tuesday, May 28. His press conference was almost as well attended as had been that of Drs. Thomas, Good, and Stock. It lasted for three hours, with Summerlin flanked by his two lawyers, James Fogarty and Arthur Hooper of Stamford, and by his wife and one of his former secretaries. The possibility of a law suit against the cancer center was openly discussed. (It was not, in the event, filed, however.)

A four-page statement was handed to the reporters. It began: "Last Thursday evening at about eight o'clock, the attorneys for Sloan-Kettering Center [sic] read over the telephone to my attorneys a statement which they said was to be issued at a private press conference the next morning. Although my attorneys and I were not permitted to be present at the press conference, we understand that the statement was, in fact, issued . . ."

In his statement, Summerlin said he had not made any effort to conceal from Good the inking of the mice, but he bitterly disputed the statements of Raaf and Ninnemann that he had known about the single-eye operations on the rabbits as early as October 8 or 9. "Regrettably, these claims are false. In the light of recent events, no one wishes more than I that the actual facts regarding the rabbits were communicated to me."

Having disposed of what he apparently considered the most damaging of the committee's accusations, Summerlin got quickly to his over-all defense. His statement continued: "My error was not in knowingly promulgating false data, but rather in succumbing to extreme pressure placed on me by the Institute director to publicize information regarding the rabbits, information which I informed him was best known to the ophthalmologists, *and* to an unbearable clinical and experimental load which numbed my better judgment to consult with the ophthalmologists rather than rely on my assumption prior to making any statements."

In telling about the change in the experimental procedure with the corneal grafts, Summerlin had earlier explained that in single-eye experiments, the cornea would be transplanted into the right eye, in double-eye experiments the cornea would go into the right eye and the fresh cornea into the left. He then said, ". . . observing several rabbits with clear right eyes and opaque left eyes, I assumed that the second protocol was being followed as that combination would have been impossible under the first [single-eye] protocol." If any single statement can be said to clarify Summerlin's approach to the science of transplantation, surely that blithe assumption that the test would show what he wanted it to show must rank very high. One is also made curious about the hectic pace of a schedule that would not permit one brief telephone call to the ophthalmologists across the street to confirm his assumption.

Summerlin followed this line of defense throughout the long questioning. He had decided that Good's pressure tactics had caused his downfall even as earlier, the pressure of surgical work at the Brooke burn center had caused his transfer within that unit.

The handling of Summerlin's accusations against Good by the press (with the exception of Barbara Yuncker of the *Post*) reflected the hallowed dictum that the other side must be heard,

but perhaps equally it reflected the journalists' dissatisfaction
over Good's bland assertions that Summerlin was a "senior
scientist" and thus did not require the close supervision he
might have accorded a graduate student or postdoctoral fellow.
Just what the disgraced researcher felt was to be gained by
smearing the man who had single-handedly lifted him out of
obscurity is not readily apparent, but the printed results served
nicely to fan the flames that had, up to that point, only scorched
the edges of the national cancer program, of Sloan-Kettering, and
of its prominent new director.

Under the headline SCIENTIST DENIES CANCER RESEARCH FRAUD
the New York *Times* reported, "Dr. William T. Summerlin, the
physician-scientist at the Memorial Sloan-Kettering Cancer
Center who was found last week by an in-house review committee to have falsified and misrepresented research findings, said
today that, although he had darkened the skin of mice with a
pen, he had not faked any results or reported any untrue
findings." Reporter Brody went on to transcribe Summerlin's
characterization of the rabbit-cornea fiasco as "an honest mistake."

She followed this with Summerlin's declaration about succumbing to Good's pressure and went on to portray the dermatologist, mostly in his own words, as being a victim of stress, the
stress being Good's insistence on results plus the responsibilities
of "heading a laboratory where 25 research projects were being
conducted simultaneously along with a great deal of administrative work that included writing numerous grant applications at
Dr. Good's request . . . research, teaching, and the sole care of
Memorial Hospital's dermatology patients."

The *Times* article also quoted Summerlin as being upset by
the "impersonal, cloistered research atmosphere" at the cancer
center, upon which he blamed the depression that, combined
with lack of sleep and the champagne breakfast, caused him
"without premeditation" to darken the skin of the mice. The article concluded with the notation that Summerlin was feeling
better under psychiatric care and still had faith in his observations.

Edward Edelson of the mass-circulation *Daily News* reported the same excuses. His editors, though, put a more accurate head on the story (SHAMED DOC BLAMES PRESSURE), and Edelson managed to remind his readers twice in the course of his story that Summerlin's excuses had already been considered and rejected by a committee of his peers. Edelson also accurately inferred that Summerlin's blaming of Good and publicity and grantsmanship pressures would amplify "shock waves through the scientific community, with many scientists describing it as an extreme example of the excesses caused by today's competition for money and headlines."

As reported in considerable detail by the *Post's* Yuncker, Summerlin claimed at his Darien session that he was overworked and exhausted by the demands of clinic supervision, consultations with other Memorial Hospital physicians about their patients' skin problems, his own skin transplant patients, and the preparation of numerous research grants.

And he even went back over the supposedly halcyon period of his work at Minnesota in his effort to show that Robert Good was the man ultimately to blame for his troubles: "I didn't leave sunny Palo Alto to slog through 30 degrees below weather in Minneapolis at five in the morning to do my toxicity assays on mice in January of 1972, you know, just for the hell of it. . . . I went because I wanted to learn immunology and because I had made an observation that I didn't understand at all—didn't know how real it might be but knew enough to know that it needed to be understood in a more fundamental fashion and dissected in the laboratory. So I'm off to Minnesota and I'm dragging my wife and three sons along and I'm entering into a Ph.D. program to boot and directing Bob Good's clinic . . . And so, on top of that, the man I'm working with at least peripherally, the man I went there to work with but whom I very seldom saw in terms of consultation on my work, gets an offer to come to New York to be director of the Sloan-Kettering Institute."

What, Good was later asked, was his relationship with Summerlin at Minnesota? He replied at some length: "It was pretty much the same as I have had with all of the fellows who have come to work with me. I treat them as if they were my own sons. When Summerlin came, I took him out to my farm and we spent several days going over plans. When I had to go away during that period, Bill and his family stayed at the farm, sort of getting adjusted to Minnesota. I outlined the experiments that I thought would be necessary and that he ought to do. I helped get him oriented to the facilities and the people. I spent a great deal of time with him in those days and also a lot of time checking his prior work. I had been very surprised that Professor Farber of Stanford was miffed at me for attracting Summerlin to Minnesota. After all, he had absolutely no grant money at all. I had to scramble around to get a fellowship for him and scrounge some money from a little pathology fund that we had for temporary support. When he said, 'I'm coming to your lab to work out my discovery,' well, I asked him what he was going to use for support, and he said, 'I'm sure you'll be able to find me some support and I don't need much,' but I was very much concerned with a guy doing that. That was unusual behavior to begin with. It was impressive but unusual. Later, of course, he was more extreme in seeking support than anybody else. Many times, just like with all the fellows, we had his wife and children out for holidays at the farm. We were very close then." Good also gave Summerlin an added vote of confidence by placing him in charge of the hospital's transplantation clinic, his duties being to make certain that proper records were kept and accurate reports made by the staff of resident surgeons and internists.

Once they were settled at Sloan-Kettering, Good had written for his protégé letters of introduction to some of the world's leading experts in transplantation immunology and had sent Dr. Summerlin to Europe to visit them, knowing well that their skepticism would be a healthy challenge to the younger man and that it would enhance his sophistication.

Things did not always work out very well, however, as was the case with Summerlin's visit to London to call upon Professor Leslie Brent at London University's Department of Zoology. Sir Peter Medawar's former colleague is not known particularly as an innovator or an experimentalist, but his critical acumen is widely recognized in the field of transplantation biology, and his questioning at international symposia has sent many an aspiring investigator back to his or her laboratory in a more humble frame of mind.

Good told about the London-New York correspondence between Brent and Summerlin: "One of Brent's major functions is policing the field and keeping out the garbage. I got a letter from Brent in the summer of '73 saying, 'Bob, I just can't communicate with your man Summerlin. He will not give me details; he will not tell me how he does things.' Brent had started trying to duplicate Summerlin's work after the transplantation meetings and so I called Summerlin in and I said, 'Hell, you've got to tell people exactly what you do. You've got to communicate with them. If you're having problems, be honest with them. Tell them you're having problems.' But I think he was too disorganized to answer Brent.

"Brent sent me a whole pile of correspondence that he had had trying to get this information. So I wrote him a letter of apology or called him on the phone and after I talked to Summerlin he apparently began communicating with Brent. But this was one of the things that angered the scientists. Nobody insists that you always be right in science. It's the method of science to establish what is right. But the rules of the game are you have to be honest. You have to report what you observe and you have to report it in such a way that others can confirm it. And those were the things that then came into question."

Toward the end of November 1973, Good had called a staff conference at which his researchers would, in ten minutes each, report their progress. Summerlin, said Good, evinced no sign whatever that all was not going well. "When he made his presentation," said Good, "I was just dumbfounded. He didn't present any of the questions that were being raised. He just presented it as though it were the same as the spring before, without any of the failures Ninnemann and Raaf were getting. I talked to him. I said, 'Gee, Bill, it's just as though Brent didn't exist, as though Ninnemann didn't exist.' And he says, 'I am absolutely convinced that these are all technical matters.' And, you know, a negative doesn't disprove a positive. There have been many examples of investigators, particularly after they have changed locations, fail-

ing to duplicate previous finding. That's why I didn't dump the
Summerlin thing in the winter of 1973."

In February 1974, though, just before the collapse of Summerlin's project, Good had brought some of his people down to the
fashionable East Fifties to the town house of the redoubtable
Mary Lasker for what he calls a show-and-tell session. The
presence of Summerlin, at this gathering, breathlessly related
to any reporters who would listen by Ruth Maier, Mrs. Lasker's
somewhat naïve publicity agent, was a chief factor in later criticism by the press of Good for continuing to push the young
dermatologist forward when he had good reason to doubt the
work. Good denies emphatically that he in any way particularly
praised Summerlin's work at the Lasker soirée. "In introducing
Summerlin, what I said was I told the story of a German patient
treated at Memorial whose transplant had succeeded, as I understood it, as it had been presented to me, and I said, 'This
is why we think that Summerlin's work, if it can be confirmed, if
it can be reproduced, may be among the most important things
in the Institute.'" (The German patient's skin graft had already
fallen off by Christmas time, but Good didn't know that.)

Summerlin's recollection of those times, as he limned the
period for reporters at his May 28 news conference, was very
different. Where Good insisted that he had only wanted Summerlin to proceed slowly and cautiously in the face of colleagues'
skepticism, the latter argued that Good was pressuring him to
make and report new discoveries. "I was brutally told by Dr.
Good that I was a failure in producing significant work. When
that started happening, I refused to believe it." Summerlin complained that the fellows in his laboratory reported not to him but
to Good. He said he missed the easy camaraderie of Minnesota
and translated his emotions into a sports metaphor. "I can't
play golf. If I hit a ball, I want someone to hit it back. I love
tennis. When I was coming here I thought, 'Wow! just think of
all those playmates.' But I couldn't get them out on the court."

Summerlin's recollection of the events of the fall of 1973 differs
in other ways from that of his mentor. "After the November all-
day lab meeting—and, by the way, I was the only director of a
laboratory that sat down with my entire staff for a whole day of

review sessions and had Bob Good invited and got all the nitty-gritty on the table where everybody could see it . . . after that long day in which we really went at it tooth and nail, and I had a ball because I thought this is what research is all about, laying it on the table and knocking heads and having fun talking about the pluses and the minuses and pros and cons, Good comes up to me and I'm thanking him and I said, 'Gee, you know, I appreciate your spending this time with us,' and he said, 'Yeah, you know, it was good to do this.' Then he said 'You know the thing that bothers me, Bill, is that you've been here for six months and you haven't really made any major new observations.' And I said, 'What?' And sort of from that point forward I think things really began to go down hill. And at some point later Rebecca said to me, 'You know, I think he just wants you to quit.' "

Summerlin also complained of his extraordinarily heavy clinical work load and the dozens of research projects he was co-ordinating with other scientists. He said he was unable to satisfy Good's lust for results, for new reportable achievements. Here his account and that of a former co-worker collide.

Summerlin's clinical research nurse, Joyce Solomon, recalled: "In our section we had a larger group of people—nurses, secretaries, technicians, postdoctoral fellows—than any other department. The purpose was to enable Dr. Summerlin to handle the combined work load of being a scientist and a clinical physician. When I first came to work for him, he had mentioned lots of projects he wanted to get into. I was very enthusiastic about it, but I realized that after almost a year we had gotten to very few of these.

"He and I just don't count research projects the same way. Some of the doctors here at Memorial consider a research project to be a very detailed collaborative study involving frequent communications by telephone, the sending of blood samples back and forth, and writing a paper with the other investigators. But I suppose you could count sending a blood sample once a month to a researcher in Canada a collaborative study. I don't think you can count the sending out of blood samples and so I don't feel that we were involved in twenty-five or thirty collaborative research studies."

Asked whether there were any clinical studies she felt were typical of the effort in the hospital and institute, Solomon replied: "There was a project in which we were studying wart viruses with Dr. Magdalena Eisinger, and occasionally we would take a wart off a patient's hand and send it over to Dr. Eisinger. That was the study. We were supposed to be doing a study with a Canadian physician on melanoma. I used to send him an occasional blood sample from a melanoma patient. Then, of course, there were the four transplanted patients that were funded with federal money. It was very difficult to find patients needing a transplant who wouldn't prefer to wait and see if their ulcers or burns healed than spend a couple of weeks in the hospital and then come back for follow-up studies. That may have thrown Bill off a little. But even with the four patients we did have, we could never seem to get an organized protocol [system for therapy] out of Bill. His methods of doing the transplants would change and he would never come out and explain to us why he was changing. One time he would use cadaver skin as a dressing and the next time he wouldn't."

The nurse also spoke of Summerlin's relations with the clinic patients. "Initially, when I first started working with Bill, we had a list of dermatologic conditions that might provide some clues as to immunology and cancer research. We saw very few such patients, and when we did, he would talk to them about future plans and new treatments but in reality none of them existed. After a number of months, though, the patients begin to ask for explanations. Their hopes had been raised and nothing was forthcoming. The clinical co-ordinators kept asking him for protocols on how to handle these patients. He would miss meetings and always have a dozen reasons why he hadn't written the protocol. He was supposed to be the leader and he did not lead. He did not produce. We had a group of patients who were being told that laboratory studies were being done when, in essence, they were not.

"The patients would call, and you can only just stall so long. To me it wasn't honest science. You don't put off someone who has a disease. They feel you are giving them hope. In this cancer hospital most of the doctors have a special sense of responsibility to the patients. Bill didn't seem to have that."

Finally, as for Summerlin's accusation that Ninnemann and Raaf had lied about telling him of the single-eye rabbit corneal transplants, Barbara Culliton, in a second long article in *Science,* pointed out, "There were two of them against Summerlin, whose credibility was seriously in doubt."

It is true, however, that in mid-November Ninnemann had gone to Good and had demanded to be transferred to another laboratory and out from under Summerlin. "Dr. Ninnemann was very agitated and upset," Good has recalled, "and he said he didn't want to work for Summerlin, that he didn't trust him, and that every time he'd make an appointment with him, Summerlin would disappear. I was very much concerned about this, and I agreed to reassign Dr. Ninnemann up to Rye."

Ninnemann remembered, "Dr. Summerlin was, throughout, friendly toward me, but I was growing increasingly impatient with him. I only had two years to spend as a research fellow, and I had already spent six months exploring what seemed to be a blind alley." Raaf, however, continued to work on the rat para-thyroid glands in Summerlin's laboratory.

What was to be gained by either Raaf or Ninnemann in telling less than the truth—or more—about when they had separately enlightened their boss about the true nature of the corneal exper-iment? In fact, their information given to the peer review com-mittee caused them enormous embarrassment owing to a misun-derstanding involving Culliton and Stock.

After the May press conference at the hospital, the *Science* writer had gone to Stock, the peer review committee chair-man, to ask why in heaven's name Raaf and Ninnemann had sat by while Summerlin continued to talk at the institute and else-where about the successful double human-to-rabbit corneal grafts. Stock simply said he didn't know, implying in a way that the two juniors had been present when such misrepresenta-tions had been made. Back at her desk in Washington, Culliton called the two researchers to ask them the same question that was bothering her. She left her number with voices at the other

end of the wire when she couldn't reach either man and asked
that they call her back. When neither did, she assumed that their
superiors had told them not to talk to reporters about the affair.
Considering the tight security at the press conference and the
close-mouthed policy the cancer center officials had been adopting
on the whole story previously, Culliton's erroneous conclusion
was not a difficult one to draw. Most junior scientists, not
having the luxury of secretaries, return phone calls on a very
hit-or-miss basis, mainly depending on whether they find on their
desks small scraps of paper left there with messages scribbled
by harried colleagues or technicians. That was the case in this
instance.

In her second article on the ramifications of the Summerlin
affair, published in Science for June 14, 1974, and based in part
on a long talk with Summerlin, Culliton wrote of the corneal
controversy: "In this case it is a matter of one man's word
against another's. Apparently neither of the research fellows got
along well with Summerlin, who was particularly at odds with
Ninnemann. Summerlin says Ninnemann was unwilling to communicate with him, going directly to Good instead. Ninnemann
says it was Summerlin who made communications impossible. It
is one of those situations that is almost impossible for an observer to figure out. However, a couple of points are clear.
Whether Ninnemann and Raaf did or did not tell Summerlin in
early October about the rabbits, they sat and listened to him talk
about the double eye transplants on subsequent occasions without saying a word. Just why they did not speak up is not at all
plain, to say the least."

As might have been expected, the implication that they had
participated in some sort of cover-up of Summerlin's corneal
folly produced anguish and ire in the breasts of the two young
scientists. They quickly fired off a joint letter to Philip Abelson,
Ph.D., editor of Science, bitterly protesting Culliton's statement,
hardly the action of two men who had told lies in furtherance of
a vendetta against their former boss. For what it tells about the
tender egos of scientists and for its commentary on Summerlin's
charges of falsehood, the letter is reproduced here as published
in Science in late August:

"It was with surprise and dismay that we read Barbara J. Culliton's report 'The Sloan-Kettering Affair II: An uneasy resolution' (News and Comment, 14 June, p. 1154). The following inaccuracies which appeared in that report call for correction. Culliton states that 'it is a matter of one man's word against another's' as to whether we informed Summerlin that only single-cornea experiments were being performed by ophthalmologists Bartley Mondino and Peter Laino. She further states that '. . . a couple of points are clear. Whether Ninnemann and Raaf did or did not tell Summerlin in early October about the rabbits, they sat and listened to him talk about the double eye transplants on subsequent occasions without saying a word. Just why they did not speak up is not at all plain, to say the least.'

"These are serious and false allegations that unfairly raise questions about our integrity and motives. The truth is that each of us, after conversations with Mondino, independently advised Summerlin that he was misinterpreting the rabbit cornea experiments. At that time he appeared to accept our corrections, and we never again saw him present rabbits that he claimed had received double corneal transplants. Another statement by Culliton—'Apparently neither of the research fellows got along well with Summerlin . . .' is also untrue and appears to be a further attempt to discredit us.

"We cannot understand why Culliton failed to interview either of us (or Mondino) prior to writing her lengthy and widely circulated account. That she should have contacted us would seem to have been required by professionalism and sound journalism. To us, this is a clear example of a science writer's publishing prematurely before she understands or has fully investigated her subject. The facts in this affair make it inappropriate to spread responsibility for Summerlin's irrational actions. Care should be taken to present these facts accurately and thus prevent damage to those who were associated with him for a short time."

The peer review committee also felt impelled to comment about Summerlin's rationality. Its May 17 report said, "The committee notes Dr. Summerlin's personal qualities of warmth and enthusiasm that have engendered confidence in himself and his findings on the part of many who have heard or met him. On the other hand the haphazard and desultory conduct of his everyday affairs entailed constant inconveniences and more serious troubles for others: repeated letters requesting scientific protocols unanswered, appointments and promises unkept, and juniors left without employment or in straitened financial circumstances. The same disarray in his laboratory organization was evidently the cause of severe frustrations among his scientific colleagues, to the point where his juniors in particular found him evasive and lost faith in him and his research."

In a letter published in the same late August issue of *Science* as that of Raaf and Ninnemann, sociologist Bernard Faber of Connecticut College gave short shrift to Thomas and others who would excuse Summerlin's conduct on the grounds of emotional upset: ". . . as [Dr. Thomas] Szasz has also argued, the reliance on such a label to explain behavior represents an abnegation of moral responsibility. . . . This raises the question of why Summerlin should be let off so easily, for he violated one of the principal mores of the profession. It seems to me that professional scientists are too quick to duck the real issue here. They seem too willing, on the most tenuous basis, to excuse the behavior of a colleague—even one who has broken their most sacred rule."

7

Legislation and Disease

THE AMERICAN PUBLIC, known to the rest of the
world as the originator of fads and fetishes, suffers from time to
time with a preoccupation over a single disease. Today that
disease is cancer. In 1878, when Congress passed the first federal
quarantine laws, we were obsessed with the dangers of yellow
fever and cholera. In 1955, when Dr. Jonas Salk was placed on a
pedestal, the nation was in the throes of poliophobia. The public's attention had been focused on infantile paralysis by Pres-

ident Roosevelt's handicap and the canny exploitation of a relatively unimportant disease by Basil O'Connor, Roosevelt's law partner and head of the National Foundation for Infantile Paralysis, also known as The March of Dimes. (With its name truncated, the National Foundation now raises funds to combat birth defects.)

The fact that cancer is today receiving a lion's share of public attention is a more complex phenomenon. To be sure, the disease will strike one of every four persons now living and will kill one in six. However, unlike cardiovascular and kidney disease, the vast majority of cancer patients who succumb to the disease do so in the last years of the U.S. lifespan, the late sixties and seventies. Also, for reasons that are obscure, cancer had almost the tabu status of a venereal disease all through the nineteenth century and well into the twentieth. And not only venereal but hereditary, thus stigmatizing the offspring of patients who died of tumors. It was not until 1922, as Stephen Strickland points out in his book *Politics, Science and Dread Disease* (Harvard University Press, 1972), that the United States Hygienic Laboratory, predecessor of the Public Health Service, started supporting a special cancer laboratory at Harvard. Strickland relates that in that year the combined in-house and Harvard outlays by the U.S. health facility for cancer research amounted to only $11,000.

By 1928, however, West Virginia Senator Matthew M. Neely was ready to take on the disease. He called for a big federal appropriation aimed at conquering cancer, and he rolled out the accustomed congressional oratory of the Coolidge-Hoover period: "The tears it has wrung from weeping women's eyes would make an ocean. The blood it has shed would redden every wave that rolls on every sea." A year earlier, the senator had decided that the remedy for cancer was a reward of $5 million to be given to the first person to come up with a cure. As the avalanche of "cures" fell upon him, Senator Neely became convinced that this approach was impractical.

Though the West Virginian didn't get the appropriation he wanted, he and his Democratic colleague Senator Joseph E. Ransdell of Louisiana managed to convince the Congress that the United States had health concerns that were just as important as infectious disease, which had been the principal target of the Hygienic Laboratory up to that point. Congress, in fact, passed a bill in 1930 establishing a National Institute of Health and endowing it with $750,000.

During the first Roosevelt administration a medical man and a congressman, both Texans, teamed up to fight for greater emphasis on cancer research in federal health programs, a campaign that had its close replica thirty years later. The issue was the same: whether or not to splinter the National Institute of Health to form an autonomous cancer institute. Dr. Dudley Jackson, a San Antonio surgeon, and a famous FDR gadfly, Representative Maury Maverick of Texas, finally succeeded in the face of bitter opposition (some of it from the American Medical Association, which then as later smelled "socialized medicine" in the cancer bill) in hacking the National Cancer Institute (NCI) out of the NIH.

An interested spectator when the NCI bill was finally signed, in 1937, was a freshman representative from the state of Washington, Warren Magnuson, who later became chairman of the Senate Subcommittee on Labor, Health, Education and Welfare Appropriations, which oversees the NIH and NCI funding. In 1974 Senator Magnuson's sub-committee approved a cancer budget that was a thousand times bigger than the $700,000 appropriated to found NCI in 1937.

Among those opposing the bill establishing the NCI was the formidable Dr. Ewing, then director of Memorial Hospital. Though he subsequently became a member of the National Cancer Advisory Panel, his comment could well have come from one of the academic opponents of the cancer bill thirty-five years later. "This solution," said Ewing, "will come when science is ready for it and cannot be hastened by pouring sums of money into the effort." Those are not the sort of words that the American Cancer Society likes to hear. The society, known then as the American Society for Control of Cancer, had pushed the original NCI bill in opposition to the American Medical Association. The cancer society orchestrates its campaign for funds carefully but with little regard for consistency. While it keeps an up-to-date list of celebrities who have died of the disease, it also encourages

articles by or about people who have survived cancer's onslaught
and publicizes the celebrities among them. In 1974, for example,
writers received for their possible use the story of a man named
James Jackson Doty who had been treated in 1970 by surgery
and radiation for cancer of his right testicle and who in the
summer of 1974 was preparing to swim the English Channel.
Shirley Temple Black's 1973 account of her mastectomy after
early detection of a breast tumor was another coup for the society, plugging as it did, the theme "Early Detection Means
Longer Life." So were Betty Ford's and Happy Rockefeller's
operations.

This slogan pinpoints one of the many ambiguities inherent in
making the public aware of cancer. It can easily be self-fulfilling
and hence misleading. Since a tumor in its earliest phase, when it
is a single aberrant cell or perhaps two or four cells, is undetecta-
ble by any medical tests known today, doctors cannot know the
moment when a person develops cancer. Therefore, two people
could become cancer victims on the same day but the tumor of
one of them might be diagnosed as cancer a year before that of
the other. If subsequently, both died on the same day, the patient with the earlier detection would obviously think he or she
had lived a year longer with cancer. So would the physicians.

It is also true that the kind of genetic change that occurs when
a cell somehow escapes the normal body control mechanisms and
sets off on its destructive, reproductive rampage plays an enormous role in determining its host's ultimate fate. Cancer specialists also know that survival often depends on the type of cell that
has run amok in the patient's body. Bitter controversies are raging over the most common cancers of older men and women. For
cancer of the prostate gland in men the argument is over
whether removal of the gland (with impotence almost the invari-
able sequel to surgery) really prolongs life in an age group susceptible to many other potentially fatal diseases. For breast
cancer, early detection and prompt removal of the tumor is best.
The argument is over how much tissue should be removed to obtain maximum survivals.

And there is the matter of defining a cancer cure. If Drs.
Thomas and Burnet are correct—if, in fact, the cancer victim

is basically suffering from a deficiency of his or her immune system—then the removal of a cancer by surgery or its destruction by radiation would still leave the patient in a situation where he would be more likely than a noncancerous person of his age to acquire another tumor. Medicine generally, and the cancer society in particular, have defined a cured cancer patient as one who survives five years after cancer has been diagnosed. This definition, of course, makes it possible for a cancer victim dying in his or her sixth year of the disease to be both cured and dead simultaneously.

Finally, there is the problem of the location of the tumor. Cancer in and of itself does not kill its victims. A patient with a brain tumor frequently dies of the pressure generated by the growing mass of cells in the enclosed box of skull. Cancer patients with small and slowly growing tumors frequently succumb to neglect while being carefully cared for in bed. Insufficient exercise can give rise to blood clots in the legs that, traveling through the veins and arteries, eventually are trapped in a lung vessel that is too small to let them pass. The patient then dies with pulmonary embolism. Since the fatality is classifiable as a cardiovascular death resulting from cancer, it is at least arguable whether those plumping for more cancer money—from the point of view of the American Heart Association at the expense of the National Heart and Lung Institute—should be allowed to claim such patients as cancer deaths to prove their case. Likewise, patients with leukemia usually succumb to an overwhelming infection or hemorrhage. Their demise could thus be linked to diseases in the domain of either the National Institute for Allergy and Infectious Disease or the heart-lung area.

Such niceties, however, are not normally of great concern to congressmen looking for a stone of disease on which to inscribe their names as a testimonial for the next election. It was again a Texan—and a liberal Democrat as well—who led the renewed cancer campaign in 1970. Senator Ralph Yarborough, chairman of the Senate's Labor and Public Welfare Committee, and his allies almost succeeded not only in further splintering the National Institutes of Health but almost in dismembering them. And he lost the Texas primary that summer anyway.

Yarborough's idea was to increase the cancer institute's budget. As a first step in that direction he appointed a twenty-six-member committee of consultants on cancer, half of them to be knowledgeable laymen, the rest doctors and scientists. To head the committee, the Texas senator chose a fellow Texan, though a transplanted one and an independent Republican to boot, Memorial Sloan-Kettering's vice-chairman Benno Schmidt. The committee barely got its report to the lame-duck senator before his term was up, but it lived up to all the cancer enthusiasts' expectations and more. Not only did the report urge a much higher rate of spending for research on cancer—that had been a foregone conclusion—but it recommended a whole new agency, a National Cancer Authority, created along the lines of the Atomic Energy Commission and the National Aeronautics and Space Administration and, like them, designed to snip excess yards of red tape away from all enemies of the nation's "implacable foe."

As Yarborough faded back to Texas, Senator Edward Kennedy moved quickly to make the issue his own. The House of Representatives had passed a resolution urging an all-out war on cancer in 1970, and Kennedy announced at year's end that he would promote legislation in line with the cancer committee's recommendations when the new Congress convened in January 1971.

It was not, however, to be expected that NIH director Robert Marston would applaud the sack of his empire that loomed with removal of its highest-priced institute and the one best known to the taxpayer. If one out of six Americans was scheduled to die of cancer, as the committee vowed, then one out of the eleven institutes was going to keep on being against cancer. The opposition of the NIH brass was predictable, but what President Nixon's stance would be was less obvious. With one eye on his unpopular though inherited Vietnam war and the other on Kennedy's high poll ratings, Nixon cut the ground from under his own budget bosses by reopening the NIH money chest and inserting another $100 million for cancer before the new Congress had even organized itself. Now the country would know who was most against cancer! And on top of the extra money, Nixon spelled out the goal in his State of the Union address in a sentence that not even the American Cancer Society writers could have improved upon. "The time has come," said the President of the United States, "when the same kind of concentrated effort that split the atom and took man to the moon should be turned toward conquering this dread disease."

Heaven knows, there was more cancer hardware already in U.S. hospitals than could be used on a daily, economic basis. You could not only irradiate patients with megavolt beams of electrons and spot a liver tumor half the size of your pinky with $100,000 radioactive scanners but you could breathe for the patients and pump their blood around long after any semblance of life remained in their brains. But in 1944 and 1961, science knew much, much more about the atomic nucleus and rocketry than doctors even now know about cancer.

The battle over the status of the federal cancer effort seesawed back and forth throughout most of 1971. On one side, pushing hard for an independent bureau freed from the layers of supervision in the Department of Health, Education and Welfare were financier Schmidt, Mary Lasker, the American Cancer Society, most cancer researchers, and two senators, Kennedy of Massachusetts and Jacob Javits of New York. On the other side were the HEW brass, Democrat Representative Paul Rogers of Florida, chairman of the House Subcommittee of Public Health and Environment of the Committee on Interstate and Foreign Commerce, and most of the nation's academic medical establishment. In the middle was the President, infuriating both sides by his seemingly uncertain stance on the legislation.

After hectic lobbying, press agentry, and arm twisting, the compromise was struck that kept the National Cancer Institute where it was but made its director a White House appointee as it also did his boss, the NIH director. The House-Senate compromise bill, the Cancer Act of 1971, was finally voted in November and the President signed it on December 23 with Rogers, Kennedy, Mrs. Lasker, and cancer society officials looking on and evidently satisfied. The bill authorized expenditures of $1.59 billion for cancer research over the next three years. It also set up a National Cancer Advisory Board that would be made up of five government officials, including the HEW Secretary and the

NIH director, plus nineteen members—two thirds of them scientists or physicians—to be appointed by the President. In addition, the bill established a three-man panel composed of one layman and two doctors or scientists that would keep the President informed of progress and administrative problems in the program that might need his attention.

This triumvirate was originally composed of Benno Schmidt, Dr. Good, then still at Minnesota, and Dr. R. Lee Clark, president of the M. D. Anderson Hospital and Tumor Institute in Houston.

While this trio would advise the President, the twenty-four-member advisory board would advise the director of NCI, whose budget would no longer be under the control of the Secretary of HEW or of the director of NIH, but of the President himself. The White House had already removed the well-liked Dr. James A. Shannon as director of NIH in 1968 and had replaced him with a more malleable executive, Dr. Marston. Now, in early 1972, the gusts of new money heading toward the National Cancer Institute seemed likely to blow away its director, Carl Baker, an old hand in NCI administration.

The hoopla over the nation's embarkation on the conquest of cancer had produced great expectations throughout the land, and the director of the NCI would have to exhibit finesse in dealing with a Congress that was giving him so much money and autonomy. Here, for example, was Representative Daniel Flood of Pennsylvania, chairman of the House Subcommittee on Labor, Health, Education and Welfare of the Appropriations Committee, questioning Baker, for whose appropriations his committee was responsible:

FLOOD: Every time the phone rings, I expect to pick it up and have you tell me that we have broken through in cancer virus research.

BAKER: I don't think it happens as a breakthrough like that.

And a little later—

FLOOD: What day are you going to tell us, what month and year, "Here, hallelujah," as you've done with polio and measles?

BAKER: I don't think it is going to come that way.

While this kind of inane dialogue was going on up on Capitol

Hill, the National Cancer Advisory Board under the chairmanship of University of Pennsylvania surgeon Jonathan E. Rhoads was holding its first meeting, and its members, too, found the climate of high expectations uncomfortable. The meeting room was jammed with more than a hundred interested observers, and one member of the board described their first, get-acquainted session as a "circus." Finally, at the suggestion of board member Dr. W. Clarke Wescoe, chairman of Sterling Drug, Incorporated, the room was cleared.

There was an immediate problem requiring definition and a strong policy from the NCI: How much of its new money was the cancer institute going to put into the prevention and diagnosis of cancer, that is, to doing better what medical science already knew how to do? Such approaches would be aimed at educating Americans as to carcinogenic environmental factors such as smoking that could, presumably, cut the cancer toll if avoided, and at making more widely available the tools of early diagnosis such as cell sampling for the discovery of cervical (uterus) and lung cancer and the new x-ray and heat-scanning methods for breast cancer screening. When Baker took his budget request to Representative Flood's subcommittee, he asked for only $430 million for NCI in fiscal 1973 and only $4 million of that sum for cancer control. The subcommittee was surprised to find an agency head coming in and asking for less—$100 million less—than that year's ceiling authorized by the recently passed Cancer Act. Evidently Baker, something of a plodder and schooled in the no-can-do miasma of Washington bureaucracy, had not taken seriously enough the President's and Congress' demands that cancer control and research get cracking.

If Baker hadn't gotten the message, it was heard very clearly by one of his younger, more optimistic, and more aggressive colleagues at the NCI. Frank J. Rauscher, Jr., now in his mid-forties, will keep on looking like a pudgy young man until his shock of black hair changes color. For a virologist with a Ph.D. and discoverer of a tumor virus, Rauscher is an engaging type who likes to talk about cancer control in cheerful tones that convey more optimism than the words he's uttering. Though his attitude promises much, his statements are carefully guarded, evidently a characteristic that favorably impressed Richard Nixon.

In choosing Frank Rauscher to take over the expanded cancer effort and replace Baker as head of NCI, the President was tapping a scientist-administrator who told *Science* magazine at the time, "I think I may surprise some of my friends in basic research." The new director, after taking his doctorate at Rutgers, came to NCI in 1959 and had isolated his virus only three years later. His timing was impeccable, for when Congress in 1964 set up a special cancer virus research program in the NCI and endowed it with $10 million for openers, Rauscher, Baker, and a third official, Louis Carrese, were set to getting the project off the drawing board. "Within six months," Rauscher has related, "the program was off and running, and I had to decide whether to stay with it or return to the lab. It was then that I chose to go into administration."

Rauscher became scientific director of the NCI for etiology (causation) in 1969 when Baker was promoted to the directorship by Marston. In that post Rauscher had favored more action in the field of environmental factors and immunology and more in widespread screening for early detection of cancer. With a $30-million ceiling set for cancer control activities under the 1971 act—an area of effort that Florida's Representative Rogers had insisted be specified in the legislation—it was apparent that Frank Rauscher would have asked for more than $4 million.

Though the presidential panel of three advisers and most of the board welcomed the appointment of Rauscher, there was one notable exception, the Peck's Bad Boy of biology and professor of molecular biology at Harvard. In the mid-1950s James D. Watson, an American, and his Cambridge University colleague Francis H. C. Crick had raced California's maverick chemist Linus Pauling to be the first to understand and describe how genetic information is inscribed in the cell nucleus. Watson's and Crick's victory, their model of the immense deoxyribonucleic acid molecule (DNA) and its mode of dictating protein formation through complementary ribonucleic acid chains (RNA), had won them a Nobel prize in 1962, along with an Oxford colleague Maurice H. F. Wilkins.

In 1972 Watson, having achieved one of molecular biology's most spectacular and fruitful advances in England with rather less money to support the effort than top American cancer researchers spend in a month, voiced his doubts about the big new program. He called the Rauscher appointment "a very sad event," after writing an article for the *New Republic* that took a dim view of the immediate future in cancer research. Watson, whose candid account of his and Crick's maneuvers to beat Pauling to the Nobel garnered many a brickbat and many a reader for his book *The Double Helix,* wrote that there were as yet no secure strategies for attacking cancer in new ways. He urged the younger biologists and biochemists to make a concerted grab for some of the new cancer money and to take it to "flexible and nonauthoritarian" laboratories where they would be free of the worn-out notions of their elders and not tempted to "grind out . . . science so that tenure will come."

But if Watson thought there was going to be more money for the younger crowd, the Nixon budget legionnaires had a message for him and all the medical centers and schools around the nation. Sure, they were going to spend more money for cancer control and cancer research, but the NIH would phase out its program of training grants and teaching fellowships. As the medical center administrators saw this maneuver, it was comparable to declaring a war on hunger and famine, appropriating millions for farm machinery and fertilizer and then cutting back on the quantity of seed a farmer could plant.

Good recalled his advocacy of the training-grant system during his year on the President's panel. He said, "I told the President first of all that the additional funding had to be add-on and not substitution, and I've said that over and over again and that's what Benno Schmidt and I spoke for repeatedly. And another thing I persistently advocated was 'Don't whatever you do turn off the faucet for the young scientists, the money that brings fellows in, because the solution to the cancer problem is in the minds of those young people.'"

Eventually, in July of 1973, the government reversed itself and, in an awkward press release that pretended to change the old policy of postdoctoral training grants, revived the system with $30 million, enough for 3,000 new grants, for a total of $90 million altogether.

When Good was heard at the White House, he also made another point. "I advocated keeping the new funds *in* the granting system with its peer review and not putting it into contract research." But the contract machinery was by 1972 deeply embedded in the cancer research works. The idea of a war against cancer, with attendant connotations of defense industries and the comparisons with the space program, where contracting had been so successfully used, lured the cancer institute into a scandalous situation. Here again, the notion of a quick success paved the way for expansion of the special cancer virus program whose contract research policies *Science*'s Barbara Culliton was already calling "controversial" back in the spring.

⌈A decade ago there were already a baker's dozen of viruses that could transform cells growing in tissue culture into a state that closely mimicked malignancy, if it was not identical. When the tumor viruses were added, the cells no longer grew in single layers, respecting each other's territoriality, but piled up in heaps. Their shape changed, too, and their nuclei took on a different appearance. Such cells, when transplanted into a suitably susceptible host animal, grew into cancers. And in other experiments, viruses were isolated from animal tumors. When these agents were injected into other animals of the same strain, they produced cancers. Was man alone immune to virus-caused cancer? It hardly seemed likely.⌋

And as Rauscher's appropriations kept going up, to almost $590 million in fiscal 1974, the special virus program also ballooned. A handful of National Cancer Institute administrators were contracting for more than $40 million worth of viruses, viral reagents (such as identificatory antibodies), epidemiology studies, and animal tumor systems. It was an uneasy situation and rife with opportunities for conflict of interest. In the ten years from 1964 to 1974, special laboratories were set up by private companies and entrepreneurs to handle the work. The Pentagon's Fort Detrick laboratory for biological warfare was turned into a tumor virus research and production area—the

Frederick Cancer Research Center—and turned over to Litton Industries to operate.

But while the virus-program contractors were enjoying their windfalls, the scientific aspect of viral cancer causation was growing in complexity. No longer did it seem likely that a single virus infecting a human being could directly produce a cancer. First came animal work that showed that sometimes a "helper" virus was required or a concomitant chemical or radiological insult. To be sure, there was some controversial but stimulating epidemiologic work linking genital infection with a herpes virus (related to the agent that causes fever sores in some persons on exposure to sunlight) to cervical cancer in women and another set of data that could prove Hodgkin's disease a transmissible virus tumor of the lymphatic system. But then along came evidence that viruses capable of causing tumors might well be comfortably ensconced in the genes of all animals and humans at birth and still other evidence contradicting the Watson-Crick dogma that DNA always dictated RNA in a one-way flow of information from the cell nucleus to its protein-making equipment in the cell cytoplasm. An enzyme was isolated both at Massachusetts Institute of Technology and at the University of Wisconsin that appeared to be able to make the supposedly dominant DNA out of the supposedly subservient RNA. Since viruses are basically bits of DNA or RNA covered by a layer or two of protein, and since a number of tumor viruses have RNA as their core, there suddenly loomed a whole new way in which viruses could insert malignant messages into the DNA genes that might sooner or later be copied out to make cancers.

What had in 1964 looked like a simple hunt for viruses against which medicine might produce vaccines, as Representative Flood was still intimating to Carl Baker in 1972, turned out to be a far more complex matter with at least three different theories competing for validation and the whole picture growing murkier by the day.

The National Cancer Advisory Board was aware of the dissatisfactions voiced by virologists at the seeming exclusivity of the National Cancer Institute's program in their field. Early in 1973 the board suggested to Rauscher that he name a committee of ten scientists to look into the project. It promptly became known by the name of its distinguished chairman, Norton Zinder, microbial genetics professor at Rockefeller University. The other nine members were Dr. Good; James Darnell, then at Columbia Presbyterian Medical Center, New York City, and now at Rockefeller University; Vittorio Defendi, of the Wistar Institute, Philadelphia; Keith Porter, University of Colorado, Boulder; James Price, Abbott Laboratories, Chicago; Wallace Rowe, virologist at NIH (NIAID); Aaron Shatkin, Roche Institute, Nutley, N.J.; Chandler Stetson, University of Florida, Gainesville; and veterinary researcher Richard Tjalma of NIH (National Institute of Environmental Health Sciences), who resigned later when he switched from NIEHS to NCI. A draft of the report of the Zinder Committee was submitted to the National Cancer Advisory Board late in November of 1973, referred back to the investigatory group and resubmitted in final form on March 19, 1974. When the Zinder Committee's report was made public in March, it became apparent how far highly reputed scientists could deviate from accepted standards of integrity when tempted to bolster their theorems and prejudices with huge sums of the public's money. The peer review system that had at least kept the Summerlin caper within limits—though obviously several million dollars had been spent in exploring its ramifications and in attempts to confirm observations that turned out to bear scanty fruit, if any—was not operating in the case of the special cancer virus project.

The Zinder Committee's thirty-nine-page report first described the scope of its investigations, reviews of annual report summaries of the various segments making up the research-production projects, attendance by certain members at solid-tumor virus segment staff meetings, a questionnaire to those scientists who had asked for materials from the contractors, and so forth. Then the report cited several justifications for the value to cancer research of a special effort on tumor viruses: "In several animal species, viruses have been shown to be directly involved in cancer causation; these include sarcomas and leukemias in chickens, mice and cats and breast carcinoma in mice. The viruses involved include both DNA- and RNA-containing types.

In addition, certain viruses, when injected into newborn animals, cause a variety of tumors later in life, although their role in natural [as opposed to specially bred] populations is less clear."

Noting that to date there is "no positive and considerable negative epidemiological evidence that cancer in man is an infectious disease" and that "no definitive human cancer virus has been isolated," the committee still felt there was good reason to go on with the research. "For one, the understanding of how known cancer viruses produce malignant change in other living forms could reveal unsuspected approaches to human cancer. Secondly, because of the complexity of some oncogenic [tumor producing] viruses and their mode of inheritance, it is possible that in an outbred population such as the human one, it will be difficult to find viral particles *per se* or a host to grow them on. Again, there is no scientific rationale at the moment why what is true for other animals should not be true of humans. Furthermore, if viruses or viral gene products are involved in human cancer, specific diagnostic, preventative and curative procedures might then be available, although even on this point we should not be too sanguine. A final point must be made. At the present time the most rapid and reproducible way to change experimentally a normal cell to a cancer cell is by infecting it with certain viruses . . . From the point of view of understanding how a transformed [cancerous] cell differs from a normal cell, viral infection confers a tremendous advantage for basic studies. The tumor cell caused by a given virus *always* presents the same immunologically recognizable changes. It may therefore be possible to determine what chemical changes in a cell are responsible for at least one cancer phenotype [the manifestation of the cell's malignancy in an animal tumor]."

The committee also sought to learn from the National Institutes of Health how much money it was spending on all virus research and how much on virus research related in some way to cancer. It found that in fiscal 1972 the nation's health research center had made about 2,000 grants with peer review that came to approximately $120 million of which "about $58 million went to studies that are in some way related to cancer." Of these, NCI had awarded 100 grants in the area of virus research amounting to $7 million while the special virus cancer program [SVCP] had spent six times as much on 131 contracts. Here the committee started to reflect the criticisms of the medical research community at large. "Clearly," the Zinder Committee report said, "the SVCP funding of viral oncology overshadows the same area in NCI as a whole and approaches the total NIH effort. However, it supports only a small fraction of the relevent scientific community." The report made it plain at the outset that the committee took a dim view of such concentration of cancer virus money in so few hands. But it had much more to say about just how this concentration of money power had been handled by the chairmen of the SVCP segments, i.e. Biohazard Control (handling unseeable agents that cause tumors is a practice fraught with potentially lethal hazards), Solid Tumor Viruses, Breast Cancer, Developmental Research, Tumor Virus Detection, Viral Immuno-Epidemiology.

Many of the men and women who run the SVCP are not run-of-the-mine NCI administrator types but scientists with international reputations. The associate director for viral oncology of the NCI is, for example, Dr. John B. Moloney, one of the first men to isolate a mouse tumor virus. (The first animal tumor virus was proved to cause cancer in fowl by the late Dr. Peyton Rous of the Rockefeller Institute in 1911.) Two other NCI officials who sit in on the monthly meeting at which new contracts are voted upon and others renewed, or, rarely, discontinued, are Drs. Robert Huebner and George Todaro, best known for their authorship in 1969 of the theory that all of us carry so-called oncogenes from birth but that these segments of our DNA are normally repressed and unable to express their lethal potential. Both have long records of high accomplishment in virology at NCI.

One of the members of the Zinder Committee, Dr. Rowe, sat in on one of the monthly meetings, presided over by Dr. Moloney for half of the day, while decisions and recommendations for half a dozen contracts were voted by the SVCP segment chairmen and vice-chairmen plus a handful of NCI administrative staffers. Dr. Rowe reported that he found a serious and conscientious attitude toward their responsibilities on the part of the decision makers and an evident willingness to change the contract patterns in limited ways and to authorize critical site visits where deficiencies seemed to dictate. But he found other aspects worrisome. One was the almost complete lack of budgetary discussion, another the lack of knowledge of the panel on certain specific projects they had before them. Said Rowe, discussing the panel's handling of a contract on Marek's disease of chickens, a cancer resembling Hodgkin's disease in humans and known to be caused by a herpes virus, "I had the strong impression that none of the segment chairmen had any first-hand knowledge of Marek's disease . . . it felt as if this contract was the only information there was on this disease."

Rowe also worried in his memo to Zinder about the fact that the contractor involved in the Marek's study, Life Sciences, Incorporated, of St. Petersburg, Florida, receives all of its income from its three contracts with the virus program. Said Rowe, "This seems to create a dangerous situation where cancelling a contract could destroy a company; any personal loyalties that may have developed could become overriding." It seemed, in short, that the sort of bail-'em-out relationship the Pentagon has had with its contractors, notably Lockheed Aircraft Corp. and Grumman Corp. in recent years, might be developing, albeit on a much smaller scale, in the nation's cancer program.

Finally, Rowe pointed out the hazards of the kind of sketchy and infrequent critical review to which SVCP contractors are subjected, in contrast to the much more exhaustive review of potential or renewable grantees: ". . . [In] several cases, the scientific justification for renewing some of the contracts was recent preliminary findings. No hard data were presented and there was no critical evaluation. Perhaps this is considered the role of the working groups [advisory teams of NCI scientists and a few outsiders appointed by the segment chairmen], but from my experience on such a group, this would not take place. This problem is probably due to the concept that the role of the contract program is to speed up the pace of research. I am sure that this lack of step-by-step critical evaluation leads to inefficiency in granting funds."

The Zinder Committee's interpretation of Rowe's comments

was simple: "The segment chairmen have too much power. The whole program is in large part primarily [*sic*] an NCI in-house operation, and those who run it are also often the recipients of large amounts of money they dispense. They tend to come from a narrow section of the scientific community and certainly were not originally selected for NCI employment on the basis of their ability to run large contract programs. When the segment chairmen decide that a particular scientific problem should be studied, usually this study is delegated to a friendly colleague . . . when the work is finished or the contractor fails to produce, understandably it becomes difficult to terminate the contract. Again, since the contracts generally involve large amounts of money, an equity is developed in the work of a particular contractor. Failure on his part leads to an attempt to prop up his program with more money instead of more appropriate phasing out or termination. The information we received indicates it is more difficult to terminate a bad contract than a bad grant."

The section dealing with possible conflicts of interest was amplified more specifically later in the Zinder report. Each contracted project, said the committee, is under the supposed supervision of an NCI project officer, a man who, evidently, more often than not, turns up to do work in the contractor's laboratory. The committee specified such "extensions of intramural activities of project officers" as those of "Dr. Robert Huebner at Microbiological Associates, Flow Laboratories and to a lesser extent the University of Southern California; Dr. George Todaro at Meloy Laboratories; Dr. Charles Boone at Meloy Laboratories; Dr. Robert Gallo at Litton-Bionetics; Dr. Stuart Aaronson at Hazelton Laboratories; and Dr. Robert Bassin at Litton Bionetics. The aggregate funding of these operations is over $10 million per annum or about one fourth of the total program."

While the committee readily conceded the creative talents of the two-hat wearers, it seemed less willing to accept their excuses that the laboratories at NCI were inadequate, government procurement policies too slow, and their pace slowed by "old fuddy-duddies."

As for the writing and allocation of the contracts to one segment or another of the program, the committee found, "We seem to have the peculiar situation of NCI staff scientists writing contracts for private industry, the monies from which are used to support their own work. These contracts go for first review to the Segment Chairmen Committee of which they are often members, and then to the working groups, which they may either chair or sit on and which often contain close friends and colleagues. NCI staff scientists also move about from one of these local contractors to another in what can only be interpreted as an effort to support these contractors."

On contract allocation to various segments: "Except for the Biohazard and Breast Cancer segments—the smallest units of the program—there is no programmatic theme within the segments. The same kinds of work are done by contractors in each of the other segments. The rationale for the distribution of a particular contract to a particular [segmental] working group has never been made clear to us; it appears to be determined by the interests of and perhaps personal relationship to a segment chairman."

While the Zinder group took pains to stress that their study was not exhaustive and, indeed, frequently anecdotal, they did undertake a simple questionnaire mailing to some three hundred scientists who had made requests to SVCP Office of Program Resources and Logistics contractors for virus preparations, antibodies to viruses to be used for identification purposes, antibodies to components of viruses, and standard cell cultures with which to inoculate viruses in animals of carefully defined genetic makeup.

The committee got two hundred responses, most of them favorable, but thought it odd that this rather simple aspect of quality control ("Ask the man who orders one") had never been used by NCI to check the usefulness to the research users of the services they were buying. Said the report mildly, "It is surprising that such feedback is not already built into the program."

The committee also found that, on occasion, the SVCP was perfectly willing to pay for the acquisition of a specific capability by a contractor (usually accomplished by hiring somebody away from somebody else at a higher salary) instead of looking for another contractor who already had the capability and wasn't using it to the fullest extent. At the same time, NCI was also

loath to provide for the expansion of a laboratory whose contracted service was in greater demand than had been foreseen.
Such a laboratory was Dr. Leonard Hayflick's at Minnesota, with
a contract up for renewal at a meeting attended by a couple of
committee members. Dr. Hayflick's contract involved testing
virus cultures for contaminating mycoplasmas, a form of very
small bacteria-fungi that live, so to speak, on the border between
viruses and the next higher forms of life but resemble the latter
more than the former. When they invade a tissue culture, they
spoil test results, and so these organisms pose a constant menace
to meaningful tissue culture research with viruses. Said the committee report: "During our attendance at the Solid Tumor Virus
working segment meeting, Dr. Hayflick, a principal investigator
[contractor] asked the committee for some guidance. He
provides the mycoplasma testing service and felt that he could
not handle more than a certain number of tests per year. He was
advised by the [working] committee to restrict his service to SVCP
contractors." Thus does the in-group solve problems.

On this topic, the Zinder committee was unusually blunt: "It
was only natural that when the SVCP was formed, a small group
of investigators was involved—an 'in group.' It now represents a
somewhat larger 'in group' of investigators. Administratively its
procedures lack vigor, are apparently attuned to the benefit of
staff personnel and are full of conflicts of interest. Because the
direct targets have become fuzzy since 1964, although the available funds have continued to grow, the program seems to have
become an end in itself, its existence justifying its further existence. In doing so, it is eroding what is good in both the grant
and contract mechanisms, a fact that may account for the widespread antipathy to SVCP in the scientific community."

On a broader note, toward the end of its report the Zinder
Committee commented, "The vision that established the program
was sound, but the underlying philosophy that the role of management of fundamental science is the same as the role of management for engineering or development when the fundamental
knowledge is available, was sadly in error. Instead of allowing
the direction of the scientific program to come from the working

scientists by opening it to all, the program appears to have been a closed operation from the start.

"Success in science is an irregular and unpredictable phenomenon. When and where important discoveries are and will be made is almost impossible to determine in advance. The goal should be to maximize opportunities."

The committee went on to make a series of recommendations that would broaden United States and foreign scientists' participation in the cancer virus program and would curb its obvious abuses and deficiencies.

Moving with remarkable speed for a government agency, the leaders of the SVCP had their answer to the Zinder report ready by mid-January, easily in time to be released to the press with the committee's criticism. It was in the form of a memorandum to former committee member Richard Tjalma, now assistant director for board and panel affairs of the NCI (no comment is required on that title) from Dr. Moloney, associate director of NCI for viral oncology and chairman of the institute's cancer virus program.

(It was relatively easy for the in-house forces to marshal their defenses because the government's Freedom of Information statutes require that any ad-hoc investigating or reviewing body such as the Zinder group give thirty days' notice of any meeting so that the government may have a designated representative present at all sessions of the committee. The government's representative at the Zinder Committee's deliberations was, naturally, an NCI man, only a phone call away from Drs. Rauscher, Moloney, Huebner, Todaro, et al.)

Thus while the rebuttal consisted of some reminders to the Zinder Committee of the requirements of United States contracts with nonfederal vendors as well as an array of numbers to show that the SVCP was not as narrowly limited as the committee insisted it was, its most frequent theme could be summarized as "But we're doing that already."

Interviewed a few months after the furor had died down, Zinder said, "I felt that in many ways the people down there in Bethesda knew exactly what was wrong and that they would try to rectify things as fast as they could once our committee had gone into operation. Right in the middle of our review, for example, they came around with a document from 'upstairs' that no contractor could any longer sit on the committee he was being reviewed by. In fact, a lot of the things that we wrote about in our final report had been changed before our draft went in. But even though the situation was changing, we felt we had to review it as we originally saw it."

Zinder also explained how and why the working groups in no way constituted critical peer review cadres: "Up until last June they were all contractors and NCI people. When the SVCP was set up, it had a focused target, to check the possible role of adeno-viruses [mostly those that cause influenza and the common cold] in malignancy. There had been isolated a characteristic antigen in tissue cultures transformed by such viruses, and the problem was to search for this marker in tumors to see if such viruses had ever been there as possible causative agents. This was a project that could be thought of as a candidate for contract work, a screening program if you will. That program, as programs will, just grew and grew. Along with that screening in the late sixties there came, I suspect, the goal of a cancer virus vaccine. This was set up as a contract program and it grew as a contract program. The working groups, as originally set up, were composed of the people who were doing the investigations as a means solely of communicating, so that everybody would know what everybody else was doing and to exchange ideas. And as the program grew, they stayed on as the working groups of a vastly expanded research effort. But they never had the essential function of a peer review group, whose meetings should be an adversary proceeding. So they became contractors—whether private companies or universities or institutes—who were giving themselves contracts."

As for the money involved, Zinder explained that though the committee found that only about 12 per cent of NCI's dollars were going into the virus contracts, if one subtracted cancer control and education money, the percentage of *research* NCI dollars going into contracts was far higher.

When NCI director Rauscher was asked about the possible

development of a cancer virus vaccine for humans, he replied, "My position has always been that vaccines are something we must strive for. Vaccines are probable. But to anybody in science it's understood that it's one thing to develop the capability of making a vaccine but then you have to prove that it's at least safe. And finally you have to have the wherewithal to prove to the Food and Drug Administration and to physicians that it's reasonable to give it a chance. So even if I had a vaccination today for acute lymphocytic leukemia—which I don't, of course —it could take at least seven years to show I had a good one. For breast cancer it could take thirty-five years. I've never felt we were going to get a proven, effective vaccine in less than ten years."

As for microbiologist Zinder, he doesn't think there's going to be any cancer vaccine ever.

8

TOAdS ANd COCKROACHES

IF RAUSCHER'S virologists are gunning their expensive technology up a blind alley, if Zinder is right and there isn't going to be any "Hallelujah, we've got the vaccine," then what hope is there that our billions of federal dollars are going to produce new and better controls for cancer? History can be instructive. Two important "breakthroughs" in cancer occurred in the 1890s.

The one that most people associate with cancer therapy came

in 1895 from a German physicist who had diagnosis in mind, not therapy, and who had, in all probability, given little or no thought to the cancer problem. The German was Wilhelm Konrad Roentgen, and his "Preliminary Communication to the President of the Physical-Medical Society of Würzburg" told of charging special metal electrodes in a vacuum tube with an electric current to produce rays—which he called x-rays—that could pierce flesh and bone as readily as light comes through tissue paper. Furthermore, said Professor Roentgen, the invisible radiation would register on a specially constructed fluoroscopic screen or on a photographic negative. Even better, like a flashbulb shining through a disc of paper towel glued to a sheet of Kleenex, the rays would be absorbed to a greater degree by denser materials and one could discriminate bone from soft tissue or, as in the case of the lung, air from water by examining the x-ray pictures.

At a stroke, Professor Roentgen had provided doctors with a means of looking into the body without slicing it open. What they would see would be gradients of density, but such differences could be crucial in visualizing a water-logged lung, a bone that was being chewed up by disease, or an enlarged heart.

Though the nature of the rays Roentgen described were not defined as three separate kinds of particles until about five years later, the new diagnostic technique was rapidly adopted by the medical profession. Too rapidly. Even before World War I physicians, both ignorant and careless in handling their new gadget, were losing hands and fingers. By the 1920s, they were losing their lives to radiation-induced cancers. But long before that, Scandinavian roentgenologists had been turning the mysterious electronic emissions against skin tumors. Today, of course, particle accelerators and radioactive cobalt have long since replaced the radium and the huge vacuum tubes that cancer hospitals had used at the turn of the century. So the great leap forward of 1895 that has both enabled doctors to find small cancers and often to disrupt them with lethal beams when they are inaccessible to the surgeon's scalpel was in no sense at all directed research. And we may hope that the next forward steps in cancer may come from just such a curious and untargeted mind as that of Roentgen.

The second important cancer discovery of the nineteenth century came in exactly the opposite way. It was made by a young New York City surgeon, Dr. William Coley, who had just seen his first cancer patient die. She was only nineteen and the young Harvard-educated doctor simply could not accept the speed with which the sarcoma invaded her body and killed her after the only treatment, amputation of an arm. That was in 1890. There were no x-rays (and even if there had been, radiation has little to offer in this and a number of other forms of rapidly spreading cancer).

Coley dug into the extensive files of The New York Hospital feverishly searching for a clue to some new form of treatment. The noted Viennese pathologist Dr. Karl von Rokitansky had commented a half century before on the fact that cancers seemed to subside when their hosts contracted tuberculosis. If Coley knew of Rokitansky's acute observation, he must also have realized that treating cancer with tuberculosis—then an incurable disease—would be a strenuous form of therapy. But he did find in the hospital records a case of recurring sarcoma of the neck that the Manhattan surgeons had been unable to fully extirpate in five separate operations. The patient seemed to have survived nonetheless. The New York Hospital chart showed that during his supposedly terminal illness, he had contracted erysipelas, had recuperated from both diseases, and had gone home.

Coley tracked him down to Manhattan's Lower East Side, made certain that the man was indeed the formerly hopeless sarcoma patient, and noted that he was alive and well seven years after he should have been dead.

A streptococcal infection, erysipelas was much more common before the era of sulfa drugs and antibiotics. Though the patient suffers chills, fever, malaise, and a very unpleasant skin eruption, erysipelas is a self-limiting disease like scarlet fever and, like scarlet fever, rarely kills anyone. Thus the disease seemed to Coley a good one to test against cancer. He got permission from his chief of service at the hospital and was instructed not to try his streptococcal therapy on any cancer patient who had any chances of surviving without it. In 1891 the technique of growing streptococci was only nine years old. Coley tried and failed several times to give a dying cancer patient erysipelas with an injection of the bacteria. In desperation he turned to the famed German progenitor of modern bacteriology, Berlin's Dr. Robert Koch, who generously supplied a culture of Group A hemolytic streptococci that succeeded where the American germs had failed.

In October of 1891 Coley finally induced erysipelas in a cancer patient. Within twelve hours of injection, the patient developed a high fever, his skin erupted generously, and his cancer vanished in less than two weeks. It turned out that Coley had neither invented nor discovered immunotherapy, as the administration of bacteria or their products is termed today. The Germans, as he learned after a search of the medical literature before reporting his successful case, had gotten there first. He found documentation indicating that in Robert Koch's homeland, doctors had induced erysipelas in at least thirteen patients with inoperable carcinoma and had seen two successes.

Reading over the German literature—and treating nine more patients with indifferent results—Coley decided he needed a different technique. The patients were, of course, desperately debilitated from the ravages of cancer, and giving them another illness was too much for most of them. They died before the beneficial effects, if any, of the streptococcal infection could become manifest. Coley tried killing the bacteria and then injecting them. No good. But he had read of work at the Pasteur Institute in Paris indicating that growing streptococci with another form of bacteria called Serratia made the germs more virulent. The youthful surgeon reasoned that perhaps the germs secreted some material that was helpful to cancer patients and that if they did, this material might be more copiously produced in combined cultures of streptococci and Serratia. Growing them together, then filtering out the living organisms, and finally cleaning up his broth as best he could, the cancer researcher injected some of this broth into a young man, the first recorded dose of "Coley's toxin," in December of 1892. The youth had a large tumor of the wall of the abdomen that had invaded his bladder. There was too much for surgeons to slice out without fatally damaging other organs. The young man was going to die after a few more months of misery. Years later he finally succumbed to a heart attack, aged forty-five. Over a period of four months, with repeated injections of Coley's toxin, the huge cancer had shriveled away, never to return.

Today, headlines would trumpet a miracle cure. But until Coley's death in 1936 there wasn't in all the world the technology to produce batch after batch of streptococcal-serratial material that would permit scientists to determine once and for all whether Coley's toxin was or was not effective against cancers, and in which types of tumors and in which patients and at what stage of the disease. In Coley's time the game was played all-or-nothing. For every success reported, skeptics could document half a dozen failures, even if they chose to believe the occasional successes of the rash innovator. And worse, there was no rational explanation for why the vaccination should work when it *did* work. Immunology was a young brat then, useful only in shots for tetanus, diphtheria, yellow fever, and a couple of other tropical diseases.

Coley's research was also overshadowed by Roentgen's work. Radiation was going to solve the cancer problem as soon as all the bugs were eliminated, so why mess around with this contaminated soup that even the revered house of Parke, Davis & Co. couldn't seem to make in any consistent fashion? Although infected with the radiation enthusiasm, Memorial's Dr. Ewing was willing to have Coley treat patients in the nation's premier cancer hospital. In 1975, thirty years and more after Ewings' death and forty years after Coley's, patients at Memorial Hospital were once again being treated with Coley's toxin, manufactured, appropriately, in Germany, by the pharmaceutical arm of I. G. Farben.

Cancer research has the infuriating characteristic of occasionally becoming most fruitful when it looks most futile. Some discoveries, which themselves proved invalid, have stimulated valuable new approaches to the problem. And some—like Coley's toxin—that have lingered in scientific limbo for decades have yet to be finally judged at all.

Before taking another look backward, we need to notice the journalistic habit of playing favorites, regardless of rationality.

Two brief examples will suffice, and I shall return to one of them at the end of this chapter.

Adorning the July 29, 1974, cover of *New York Magazine* were the earnestly bearded faces of two cancer researchers in their forties, Frank Friedman and Lawrence Burton, both Ph.D.s. Above their heads ran heavy type that read "The Politics of Cancer," and just to his right and out of Friedman's line of vision came the explainer lines, "Why won't the medical establishment pay attention to these two men?" Science writer Alan Anderson, Jr., had gone out to Lake Success on Long Island, a few miles from New York City, and had watched over a period of forty-five minutes while an injection of a blood fraction melted away a mouse mammary tumor. His questions were obvious once he had seen the mouse cancer cure demonstration: Why isn't the government supporting these two men? Why do they have to get their money from Lionel Teicher, "a Great Neck businessman"? And why isn't the Memorial Sloan-Kettering Cancer Center, only fifteen lousy miles away, interested?

Together with this article lauding Burton and Friedman's continuing fight against the establishment and holding out to readers the possibility that a cure for cancer was being squelched because of jealousies and "politics," there came a boxed feature, also by reporter Anderson and headlined WHEN LABS BECOME PRESSURE COOKERS. Here, after noting that William Summerlin "blackened the skin of eighteen mice," Anderson asked the Lake Success scientists how they rated the Summerlin affair. Said Burton to Anderson, "Summerlin was overfinanced. He had to produce to justify all the money he was getting. We have to produce practical results just to survive." That quotation leaves hanging in the air two questions: what is a "practical result?" Is it curing specially bred mice of breast cancer? And second, what level of support should a cancer researcher enjoy?

The other article appeared in *Science Digest* for September 1974, headlined THE CANCER RIP-OFF. The author of this piece, Lee Edson, an experienced hand who frequently writes for the Sunday New York *Times Magazine,* was taking a cue from the Zinder report. But when he turned his attention to the search for new avenues of approach, he chose as his target Robert Good, who, he said, "has decided to investigate such discarded and scientifically unfounded 'cancer cures' as Coley's toxin (a mixture of bacteria and virus), which was developed at the turn of the century."

A word is appropriate here to point out that Edson, in his zeal to discredit Good or Sloan-Kettering, or both, made Coley's toxin sound like a health-food faddist's new vitamin. There were, in fact, no bacteria in the brew, and viruses have never been involved at all. Furthermore, the fact that radiation therapy for cancer was "developed at the turn of the century" has not damaged its acceptance by the medical establishment. It is alive and well, if not accomplishing all that its devotees claim. Good and Sloan-Kettering may expect too much from immunology in the war on cancer and may well have put too many of their eggs in one basket. The final score, however, is not yet in.

Like *New York Magazine's* Anderson, Edson, too, had a favorite disregarded cancer lead to plug. His choice was a factor isolated from the livers of sharks more than fifteen years ago and upon which Dr. John H. Heller was expatiating to this writer in 1960. Just as Burton and Friedman left St. Vincent's Hospital in Greenwich Village to found their institute in Lake Success, Heller had left Yale in 1954 to found his New England Institute for Medical Research in exurban Ridgefield, Connecticut. Heller was interested in the reticuloendothelial system and its role in cancer. The term is shorthand for a series of reactions that involve the permeability of blood-vessel and capillary walls, along with the immune systems previously discussed.

The factor Heller extracted from sharks he named "Q–10" and even managed to get tested against some terminal human breast tumors at Yale-New Haven Medical Center. Edson called attention to the fact that the National Cancer Institute had been unwilling to advance the sums that might enable Heller to analyze Q–10 and then, possibly, to synthesize it or obtain it by some more sophisticated isolation process in a purer form. Yet, it must be said, Heller is far from starving in a garret in Ridgefield. His modest laboratory there has been in business for more than fifteen years. Without judging the merits of Q–10, it seems fair to ask how much donated money has flowed through Heller's hands during this period and why he hasn't got something more to show for it than a gripe against NCI. Coley's toxin is in far better shape than Q—10, and for the reasons that we'll look at a little later in this chapter. Heller, Burton and Friedman have not been indulging in quite the now-you-see-them-now-you-don't antics of Summerlin, but it should be clear by now that all of us in science writing can be sold stories by some persuasive and articulate cancer researchers impatient with the rather plodding pace at which their peers seem to prefer to confirm supposed advances. (Like my colleagues in the field, I have frequently left a press conference at which some dazzling medical feat has been detailed by a physician only to be asked, or asking, the odd question: Do you think this guy is for real? Every reporter copes with the problem as best he or she can, but confusion is frequently the result.)

The confusion, however, is not confined to science writers. It was also apparent in a belated decision by the Nobel prize committee in 1927. The prize in physiology or medicine for 1926 went to Johannes Fibiger, who received his $32,000 almost as an after-thought by the committee. The group was in session to award the 1927 prize. Fibiger was professor of pathology at the University of Copenhagen. Copenhagen is the capital of Denmark, a country in close proximity to Sweden where Alfred Nobel made a fortune manufacturing explosives that undo physiology, if not medicine. The coveted Nobel, when awarded to Fibiger, did not come unattended by protests from scientists. The pathologist, however, defeated his critics by dying at sixty-one, only three months after he cashed the Swede's check.

Fourteen years earlier, it had been shown that radiation would induce tumors in both animals and humans. By 1918 Dr. W. E. Caldwell, Dr. C. L. Leonard, and Dr. M. K. Kassabian had all died of an occupational disease of enthusiastic physicians, radiation-induced cancer. In 1913 Fibiger was looking for other ways in which cancer could be stimulated. While examining the cancerous stomachs of some wild rodents, he chanced upon parasite larva infesting their bellies. The Danish researcher attributed the gastric cancer of his rats to the parasite's metabolic by-products, its excreted wastes. The rat tumor was named "Spiroptera carcinoma," a coinage combining the scientific names for cockroaches and their parasitic worms. The parasites originally infested the large insects and only arrived in the rodent's bellies when the rats dined on fresh cockroach. By 1927, nobody much believed Fibiger. Scientists had been feeding cockroaches to rats for years with no appreciable results in terms of tumors, gastric or otherwise. Like Summerlin's transplants, the Spiroptera carcinoma of rats could not be confirmed, and there was beginning to be a smell. By the time the Nobel committee had deodorized Fibiger's reports, however, a Japanese researcher, encouraged by the Dane's work, had found a highly reliable means of producing both benign and malignant gastric tumors in rats. He deprived them of vitamin A. Fibiger's cockroach worms might have been doing that too, but nobody ever bothered to find out once Fibiger had been honored and died. Also, heartened by Fibiger's work, another team of Japanese scientists started painting the ears of rabbits with coal tar chemicals in an attempt to induce tumors chemically. They were also rewarded with success but not with the Swedish magnate's prestigious prize.

During the same period in which controversy raged over Fibiger's claims, another scientist was driven to suicide by accusations that his data were faked. Paul Kammerer shot himself in the head on a mountain path near Vienna just a year before Fibiger received his Nobel. Kammerer's career and tragedy are recounted in Arthur Koestler's *The Case of the Midwife Toad* (Random House-Vintage Books, 1971).

The ways in which a scientist's integrity or intelligence can be impugned are legion. But the degree to which the mistaken, embarrassed, or faking researcher will suffer depends in large measure on how much emotion is being pumped into the controversy he has set off. In Kammerer's case, the bitter conflict between the disciples of Darwin and those of Lamarck had been waxing steadily more acrimonious for half a century. The essence of Lamarckism was that camels, for example, forced to conserve water by living in the desert, could, over a period of time, pass their adapted physiology on to their offspring.

Darwin attributed evolution to random mutations in the genes, leaving no room for progress based on experience or social or environmental causes.

When Kammerer switched two species of salamanders to each other's environments in 1909 and reported that in a couple of generations the animals inherited changes in their neonatal development and in their coloring, he had not intended to shore up the Lamarckian heresy. When he later went on to work with Alytes, the midwife toad, and showed development of the creature's hand webbing in response to mating in water instead of on land, Kammerer was the first to point out, as any good scientist should, that the changes in the toads could be explained as a reversion to an earlier state, one in which genes already present in the animal were encouraged to express themselves by an environment that could, presumably, effect their activity hormonally or in some other way without *changing* their genes at all.

Only a few years ago, scientists in Great Britain delicately extracted the nucleus from a fertilized frog's egg and replaced it with a nucleus from a frog's somatic (normal body) cell. Since the genetic information to make a whole tadpole is present in the nucleus of every cell in the frog, it seemed that under proper stimulatory conditions the genes might be turned on and off in their proper sequence to make a duplicate of the frog from which they were taken. And that is precisely what happened under the influence of the extranuclear control substances in the egg. Perhaps the most important point about Kammerer's tragedy is, after all, that his Neo-Darwinian enemies could not tolerate the data he presented even though he had not intended and did not claim that his work provided proof of Lamarck's ideas.

A repetition of the midwife toad episode of the 1920s seems unlikely. But there was an episode at a major Middle Western university in 1964 that bears a remarkably close resemblance to the Summerlin affair. It concerned not cancer but heart disease research and a particular enzyme. Like Good, the head of the large laboratory working on enzyme problems had invited a professor I shall call Fraley from another institution to spend a few years as a visiting professor. The researcher, in this case, had his own fellowship money from a granting institution.

Soon Fraley had isolated an important new compound and

published a communication to that effect. But when other groups at other laboratories failed to isolate the substance, the laboratory chief invited a scientist I shall call Brown from still another institution to come to his center and work out the problem with visiting Professor Fraley.

Here is the description of what then occurred, in the words of the laboratory's chief:

"Although Fraley had assured me that everything was in readiness for Brown's visit, and that active material was available, he failed to produce anything when Brown arrived. I was disturbed that what he told Brown and what he told me in the way of explanation did not correspond. My suspicions, which were latent, were then thoroughly aroused, and I examined Fraley's notebooks for the first time together with some of my colleagues. It was immediately obvious to me that the experiments in his notebooks provided no basis for any of the claims made in his two publications. I then terminated his stay at the institute and shortly afterward made a statement at the meeting of the Federation of American Societies for Experimental Biology in Atlantic City, which, in effect, denied the reliability or authenticity of Fraley's data on the basis of his actual notebooks.

"Afterwards, I became aware that this was not the first such episode for Fraley. There were several instances in his previous career of dramatic claims that others could not confirm. The pattern of deception apparently went all the way back to his graduate school days at the California Institute of Technology.

"Fraley was a charming and very knowledgeable person. He had a broad knowledge of the field and was very competent in the laboratory. He gave the impression of a very principled, thoroughly honest and modest investigator. Knowing him as I did, it was inconceivable to me that he would be anything but scrupulously honest and reliable. When I suggested controls, he would do them at once and report the results to me. Everything in the development of his work was internally consistent. It was only when the actual notebooks were examined that it became apparent that the whole story was a fabrication."

Curiously, despite the matter-of-fact recitation provided by the laboratory head, a letter of inquiry to Fraley produced a

complete denial of fraud or fakery, only an admission that his in-
experience with animal cells—he had worked with plants previously—had led him to make errors that he readily admitted
when his work could not be confirmed. "While I was a guest in
the laboratory, I found that I could not reproduce results that I
had obtained earlier. I immediately announced this failure, together with a statement that I no longer considered the results
valid in a communication to the Federation of American Societies for Experimental Biology." To back up his statement, Fraley
sent along a reprint of a paragraph from the federation's proceedings for that year. The notice, however, says only that his
data was retracted, not by whom. I have since spoken with a scientist who was present at the session in question and who in-
forms me that it was Fraley's boss who, in icily controlled tones
and with a grim face, made the public retraction. Fraley must
have forgotten that part.

Fraley also blames the lab chief for "malicious gossip" and
cited a lengthy list of the scientist's retractions, mentioning his
quarrels with colleagues and examples of malfeasance. There is,
evidently, a point at which the relationships among scientists
become very unscientific.

Memorial Sloan-Kettering's Thomas and Good may take some
comfort from the experience of the enzyme fraud since it obviously did not involve any crash program against anything
and the alleged perpetrator was in no immediate need of grants
or funding. The director of the Middle Western laboratory had,
however, one further comment. After observing that attempts at
fabrication at a major research institution are invariably doomed
to failure and thus constitute a form of professional suicide by
the faking researcher, he wrote: "I suspect that there are many
more attempts at deception than are publicized. Either they are
too trivial to report, or it becomes too difficult to prove, or, more
importantly, it is deemed too dangerous to make such accusations.
The accuser is generally blackened with the accused. The more
usual attitude toward such practices is 'Why rock the boat? Get
rid of the man and say nothing.'"

Unfortunately, saying nothing provides no guarantee that the
culprit will also say nothing. But there exists another way in

which leading research institutions can get stuck on a tar baby, as Br'er Fox did in the famous tale of Uncle Remus. The July 1974 *New York Magazine* article on Burton and Friedman already alluded to gives a piquant illustration of the problem as it relates to seeming "breakthroughs" in cancer.

After reviewing the immunologic deficiency theory of cancer causation, the author of the article, Alan Anderson, chose to ignore the laborious investigations of human immunology that started with Southam's work and have progressed to numerous attempts to cure patients both by passive transfer of immunologic components from normal volunteers and patients recovered from their cancer as well as by active immune stimulation provided by Coley's toxin, BCG, killed leukemia cells and other agents. Burton and Friedman's mouse experiments are regarded by Anderson as a major advance over immune experiments "in test tubes, an unnatural environment."

The story begins when the two scientists took their Ph.D.s in zoology at New York University and began to work on tumors of the fruit fly drosophila, best known for its highly visible chromosomes and the classic genetic breeding experiments of the late Thomas Hunt Morgan at the California Institute of Technology, for which he won the Nobel prize in medicine in 1933. It was also at Cal Tech that Burton and Friedman succeeded in isolating a factor from drosophila tumors that would induce similar cancers in other flies when injected into them at the larva stage. The instigation of cancer in so short-lived an organism as the fruit fly offered the promise of a rapid assay system, an insect model in which possible tumor factors from higher forms of life could be checked out and their carcinogenic potency possibly quantitated.

Moving to St. Vincent's Hospital in New York in the late 1950s, the two researchers were housed there by Dr. Anthony Rottino, then well known for his research on Hodgkin's disease, and were financially supported by the Damon Runyon people and the NCI. In those days there was a third member of the team, Robert L. Kassel, Ph.D., now at Sloan-Kettering. (Since Kassel has little use for Burton or Friedman now, he escapes mention in the Anderson article, though his name is on the first

mouse reports given by the trio at the New York Academy of
Sciences in 1962.)

Burton, Friedman, and Kassel centrifuged and dialyzed serum
and tumor fluids from mice and men, added them to fruit fly larvae, but did not succeed in producing drosophila cancers. They
did find that some of the five factors they were investigating
killed the larvae and others did not.

As Anderson relates, the possibility of a new, rapid screening
test attracted the attention of Sloan-Kettering scientists, and one
of them, Dr. John J. Harris, was posted off to check out the work
of the Greenwich Village workers and see what factors they were
obtaining and how. Harris told Anderson he was simply a spy
dispatched by Big Brother on Sixty-eighth Street to ferret out
the techniques of Burton, Friedman, and Kassel, and he says he
felt that was wrong. He evidently made contributions to the work
because his name appears on one of the 1962 reports in which
the group said they had isolated from both human and mouse
serum factors that would induce and factors that would dissolve
tumors.

Harris told me that he feels the group "pioneered" immune
therapy. Kassel says Sloan-Kettering offered the St. Vincent's
team a contract that would have supported further investigation
of their work and that he voted for it but was outvoted by Rottino, Burton, and Friedman. Since such contracts are usually
offered in the research field with miles of string attached, there
rarely occurs between independent medical research institutions
the kind of selfless co-operative support the public imagines to
be the rule in such dealings.

In the ensuing decade, while Burton and Friedman stuck to
their mouse tumor and serum extracts, Harris left Sloan-Kettering, partly as a result of an argument over primacy of authorship
on the Burton-Friedman-Kassel-Harris paper, and Burton and
Friedman left Rottino, evidently with few regrets on the latter's part. No further papers were published by Burton and
Friedman, now ensconced in their Lake Success laboratory,
though they indicated to Anderson that some would be forthcoming now that they "have discovered a second, more powerful
tumor-killing substance, as well as a second and perhaps a third

blocking substance." The Burton-Friedman theory, like others in the immune field of cancer research, postulates good substances in the blood that are counteracted by bad factors and also claims as perfected a method of profiling animals and people from blood tests to show whether they are normal, suffering unseen tumors, or just extrasusceptible.

If you talk to Burton, and if you ask him why he doesn't publish and why the mouse mammary tumor disintegration remains his single demonstration that the system works, you obtain little enlightenment. He had obviously implied to Anderson that the technique was ready for human trial: "What can Friedman and Burton do for a patient whose profile indicated incipient cancer?" Anderson asked in his article, and he answered that with what he had been told at Lake Success: "Legally, their hands are tied. Because they are Ph.D.s and not M.D.s, they cannot even touch a patient themselves. They are also hung up on the F.D.A. requirements for an L.D.-50 before any clinical trials can be run. L.D. stands for lethal dose and L.D.-50 means that researchers must demonstrate how large a dose of their therapeutic agent is capable of killing 50 per cent of a population of test animals before it can be judged safe for humans."

Anderson was told that mice would die of water accumulation from the size of the injection needed to give enough factor to produce any deaths at all. In fact, there appear to be two factors now involved. "What we have learned," Friedman told Anderson, "is that . . . three fractions [from serum] must be in balance to maintain health. In a normal mouse, tumor growth seems to be prevented by a tumor attacker [which he had earlier described as a peptide chain, in short, a small piece of protein]. In a mouse with cancer, we find that fraction 2 (chemically undefined) is blocking the attacker. By adding fraction 3, the de-blocker, we can free the attacker to do its work once again. If we add extra attacker, we can really put the tumor away, as you saw."

The first thing to be said about this remarkable analysis of the cancer problem based solely on findings from a special strain of mice (the C3H) that is exquisitely susceptible to breast tumors, is that it closely resembles meticulously documented and thoroughly published work of Drs. Karl and Ingegerd Hellstrom at the University of Washington, Seattle. The main difference is that the Hellstroms have been looking at the blocker as an antibody, a form of gamma globulin. The Hellstroms have been trying to sort out the role of what they term "blocking antibody" in human cancer patients and in successful and unsuccessful transplants and they have made no claims for curing anything. The Hellstroms, too, by the way, think there are deblocking factors in serum, but they are not jumping on the Food and Drug Administration for its rigid rules. They are also steadily publishing their methods and results.

"More awkward still," says Anderson, "they must do an L.D.-50 on a second species of test animals, and because other test animals are larger than mice, even larger injections would be required. Burton guesses they would have to take three months away from their work to isolate enough fraction for such tests." It is not made clear what "work" they would have to take time away from that could be more important than demonstrating some effectiveness of the fraction and its safety for, say, dogs or cats with natural cancers.

There are also at least two forms of animal cancer now known to respond dramatically to injections of normal serum from other animals of the same species. Dr. William Hardy of Sloan-Kettering, the scientist who conclusively showed that cats can infect other cats with lymphosarcoma, a disease very like leukemia in children, has also proved that an evident lack of an immune factor in a cat with a spontaneously occurring natural lymphosarcoma (not an animal that has been bred to susceptibility, as the C3H mice have been) can be countered by giving the animal serum from a normal cat. Hardy says that not all lymphosarcomas of cats can be treated in this way, but he observed that the response of the cancer can be very rapid. It may start to recede dramatically in from two to ten days.

There is also a mouse leukemia, this time in the in-bred AKR strain, that shows the same dramatic response to injections of plain, untreated serum from normal mouse strains. In this case, the researchers know that the mouse lacks a particular element that plays a crucial role in the recognition and attack of the white-cell immune system against the tumor cells.

Thus scientists now know of at least two ways in which dramatic melting away of tumors can be achieved without any abracadabra of three fractions or blockers and attackers or any of that. And furthermore, some comparable approaches have been tried in human cancer patients with a notable lack of success. The idea that Burton and Friedman are being deprived of their privilege of testing a system—proven only in one strain of mice—against tumors or tumor susceptibility in humans is simply ridiculous, L.D.-50 or no.

When I spoke to Burton, this very point came up. He complained that to prove effectiveness to the Food and Drug Administration one has to show regressions of transplanted tumor systems as opposed to the spontaneous cancers of the special mouse strains. "I don't want to spend nine months of my life learning a new tumor system," said Burton. Furthermore, FDA wants enhanced survivals of the treated animals to prove efficacy, while Burton and Friedman rely on tumor shrinkage and destruction to prove their case.

When I asked about the publication problem—why they didn't lay out their methods in print for anyone to read and try to duplicate—Burton seemed to feel that others would not be able to do the serum fractionations correctly and poor results would ensue that would set their work back. He did promise that he and his colleague would teach anyone the technique who was willing to spend three weeks learning it in their laboratory.

My next stop was Dr. Good. Why, I inquired, would it not be a good idea to send a postdoctoral fellow out for a three-week stay at Lake Success? If the Burton-Friedman offer was hedged with all sorts of conditions, such an acceptance would smoke them out, would it not? What did Memorial Sloan-Kettering stand to lose, devoted as Good has declared it to be to the investigation of any and all forms of immunotherapy?

Good replied that he was indeed interested in the Burton-Friedman serum fractions but he felt it wisest to proceed with extreme caution—". . . since efforts in the past to do this are alleged to have been frustrating, it will be necessary to do it in just the right way so that a real yes-or-no answer is obtained."

Another member of the Sloan-Kettering staff, though, provided

additional insight. "Suppose," he offered, "we do send somebody
out there to check it out. The first thing you know, those two will
be running around telling the world Sloan-Kettering has bought
their claims. That wouldn't be too good, now, would it?"

Such are the emotional factors that cloud cancer research
issues. To be an outsider is to cultivate paranoia. To be of the
Establishment and high on its roster seems to engender other
hobgoblins.

The waters of public understanding are frequently muddied
with honest mistakes that are widely publicized. Two noted
researchers at Roswell Park Memorial Institute in Buffalo had assigned a junior to work on a promising anticancer substance a
few years ago. The results of his work in cultured cancer-cell
kills were impressive, and they were in the process of writing a
report on the promising new drug when they decided to make
one final check on their subordinate's work. The senior investigators found that sloppy control of contamination had allowed
micro-organisms to enter the cultures and that it was these that
were producing the nice results.

The most recent instance of embarrassment along these lines
came in 1974 to Dr. Albert Sabin, developer of the attenuated
(live) virus vaccine against poliomyelitis. In recent years, Dr.
Sabin, working in Rehovot, Israel, at the Weizmann Institute of
Science, had turned his virology talents to cancer research, teaming up with Dr. Giulio Tarro of the University of Naples. Dr.
Andre Nahmias of Emory University in Atlanta and others have
developed some impressive statistical evidence for the involvement of herpes viruses in the production of uterine cancer, and
there is a suspicion that cancer of the male prostate is similarly
involved.

In 1973, after six years' work, Sabin and Tarro issued a blanket
indictment at a well-publicized conference in Washington, D.C.
The researchers claimed they had excellent evidence that the
herpes viruses that cause cold sores and genital lesions also
played a role in cancers of the lip, mouth, nose, throat, kidney,
cervix, bladder, and prostate. The research was based on their
finding of telltale antibodies to herpes virus in patients with those

tumors but not in people suffering other forms of cancer nor in people entirely free of the disease.

As is customary with any sweeping claim such as Sabin's in the field of cancer virology, there were many who were quick to doubt and criticize the implication that herpes virus had now been found guilty of half-dozen human cancers. In the fall of 1974 Sabin announced his retraction. And to anyone who remembered his duels with Jonas Salk over the merits of live versus killed polio vaccine, Sabin's retraction was a moment to be savored. He published a report in *Proceedings of the National Academy of Sciences* that said he had been unable to duplicate the results he had announced. Said Sabin, "I've been a scientist too long not to do that. If I find something that a colleague and I have reported that I cannot confirm, it's my duty to report it."

This, of course, does not mean that Sabin, Nahmias, and others are wrong and herpes goes back to being only a fever-sore virus. It does show that honest mistakes are frequently made and must then be gulped down in a mouthful of crow.

9

THE MONEY bUSH

VARIOUS PRIVATE FUND-RAISING operations are going
on in medical centers all over the United States, especially in the
score of cancer centers supported in large part by the National
Cancer Institute. Nowhere is the quest more urgent than at Memorial Sloan-Kettering, where a deficit of about $4 million for
1973 had grown at the end of 1974 to a frightening $7-million
gap between expenditures and income. The major contributor to
this 40 per cent increase in the deficit on a total budget of

$84,750,000 was the Sloan-Kettering Institute which, according to knowledgeable insiders, was being run as if its formally adopted budget for the year did not exist.

The budget had called for total institute expenses of $17,975,982. Of this sum, about $11.5 million was to come from the NCI, the old 47–53 ratio having been thrown away as the national cancer program burgeoned. Another million was counted upon from other government agencies, principally the old Atomic Energy Commission, which aided the operation of Sloan-Kettering's cyclotron and attendant research with radioactive isotopes. Publicly supported philanthropic agencies were expected to provide another million, trust and investment income almost $2 million more, which left about $2.5 million to be contributed to Sloan-Kettering by individuals, corporations and foundations.

As the fiscal experts at the cancer center saw the picture, this might have left a manageable deficit for the institute of under a million dollars. But Dr. Good had not come all the way to New York from Minnesota to scrimp and pinch pennies. The fiscal people watched in dismay as a combination of huge energy cost increases, salary raises, the hiring of a score of unauthorized people, and the purchase of supplies, drugs, expensive immunologic reagents, animals, and equipment, pushed the Sloan-Kettering budget into a pool of red ink—about $3.8-million worth—that was bound to leave the trustees gasping.

Furthermore, much of the money that Good was supposed to bring with him from Minnesota had not materialized. In mid-summer 1974 Charles Forbes, vice-president for development (fund-raising), had been exuberant over Good's new programs at the institute. Forbes was saying that a good proportion of the $3 million in funding Good had at Minnesota would, one way or another, end up on Sixty-eighth Street. That didn't happen, but the institute went on spending as if it had.

To see how easily a project or two can torpedo a budget, consider a proposed Sloan-Kettering research program on breast cancer to be undertaken with an eye to possible virus causation and the immune response of patients. Toward the end of 1974, one such was submitted to the NCI for funding. The expense for one year for this one project, involving co-ordination with some African researchers, was projected at more than half a million dollars. A sampling of items: glassware, $35,000; blood donors, $2,000; one clinical co-ordinator spending one fifth of his or her time, $6,000; three research associates, $54,000; electron microscope, $50,000; animal maintenance, $5,000; tissue culture media and serum, $25,000; African shipments, $5,000; ten technicians, $100,000. From this selection out of an expense sheet detailing twenty-seven separate items, it should be easily seen how taking on even a few extra research proposals can decimate a cancer research institution's budget.

During 1974, the year in which Sloan-Kettering expenditures had jumped from an anticipated level of just under $18 million to well over $21 million, the nation, as everyone was painfully aware, had experienced double-digit inflation. Just to keep pace with the 1974 costs, therefore, would have required a budget of almost $24 million for 1975. This was not in the cards. Good received word in mid-November that the 1975 budget would be about $22.5 million and would thus require cut-backs of about 10 per cent across the board. (For comparison, the research budget of Roswell Park Memorial Institute in Buffalo, which is supported in part by the state of New York, was $7.3 million in 1974; that of the newly organized Hutchens Cancer Center at the University of Washington, Seattle, was $7.2 million; and the NCI had in the fall of 1974 just awarded $1.2 million to the brand new cancer center at Mount Sinai Medical School only two miles from Sloan-Kettering in New York as start-up money based on a proposed budget of $1,750,000.)

It was at this point in late 1974 that sympathy for Bill Summerlin began to surface among Good's antagonists at the institute. They looked around and saw, or thought they saw, scientists with fifteen and twenty years of experience at Sloan-Kettering, with outside research grants of their own, forced to curtail projects while Good continued to dole out largesse to the favored few immunologists, many of them only recently arrived from Minnesota. "I can't see," remarked one disgruntled veteran, "why, if I have, say, $90,000 in outside grants and $10,000 support from the [Sloan-Kettering NCI] grant, I should

be cut the same amount as some guy who has only three publications to his name and who's getting $90,000 from this in-
stitution and has scraped up $10,000 on the outside."

Good's answer to such charges is simple. In 1976 all Sloan-
Kettering scientists will be expected to earn their keep through
grants. The single-instrument money will have been phased out,
to be replaced by perhaps $5 million as a core grant intended for
support of all institute projects, a kind of purse from which to
draw overhead expenses. At that point, a scientist without grants
of his own will simply be out of money, if not out of a job. Good
insists that this rule will apply to his recruits from Minnesota
with equal stringency. It is well known around the institute,
however, that, as was the case with William Summerlin originally, the SKI director always has a few hundred thousand
dollars from a variety of benefactors that can be pressed into service for promising studies. Given the director's current outlook
on areas of promise in cancer research, those scientists with immunologic interests are likely to be the beneficiaries of his favors.

Thus after a decade of insulation from the rigors of grant competition, the researchers of the Sloan-Kettering Institute found
themselves back in cutthroat competition with those in academic
centers and, as well, with scientists in more than a dozen newly
funded cancer centers around the nation. One former vice-
president of Sloan-Kettering, a man with more than a score of
years in basic chemical research on cancer processes, simply quit
in disgust. Others hastened to get their grant requests in circulation. But the mood of many was far from jovial. Said one of the
Summerlin escapade, "I almost don't blame him even though
what he did was crazy. Good's just leaning too hard on everybody to produce."

Worry over a new entrepreneurial approach to cancer research
funding was by no means confined to the Upper East side of
Manhattan. In January of 1975 the New York *Times* carried a
piece on its "Op-Ed" (opposite-editorial) page by Dr. Ernest
Borek, professor of microbiology at the University of Colorado
Medical Center and a noted molecular biologist. After observing
that the atmosphere in many laboratories had changed drastically with the infusion of huge sums of federal money into

research, Dr. Borek went on to comment, "Ambitious young scientists in large laboratories become especially tempted because often they are not properly supervised. As large grants for medical research become available, entrepreneurial ability in some cases was added to scientific ability in securing funds, laboratories and research associates. The researcher became an employer." Since Dr. Borek's essay was titled "Cheating in Science" and since he had mentioned the unhappy episode at Sloan-Kettering in his first sentence, it was hard not to conclude that Borek was echoing the charges of the older Sloan-Kettering men. One of them put the matter to me even more strongly. The virologist, sputtering mad, said, "I have some advice for young researchers in biology. Stay out of cancer research because it's full of money and just about out of science."

But the money, just three years after former President Nixon had signed the Cancer Act, wasn't all that abundant. The House and Senate conferences on the budget for NIH had settled on $691.6 million for the National Cancer Institute just before adjourning. However, the state of the national economy made it clear that President Gerald Ford was going to ask some major cut-backs of the new Congress. Those in charge of the cancer program found it only prudent to hold down cash disbursements in the 1975–76 fiscal year until they could determine whether substantial pruning might be asked of and accepted by the legislators. The grants request machinery at Sloan-Kettering that was being geared up in the summer hummed busily in the second half of 1974 so that by year's end no fewer than seventy-five separate requests had been approved by NCI, private health agencies, and private philanthropies. The bulk of these, of course, were approved in Bethesda, but NIH money is more evanescent than that from, say, the Rockefeller or Kresge foundations. Rauscher's lieutenants were approving bushels of grants while at the same time notifying the recipients that they would be only partially funded until the federal budget was finally determined.

Thus two of the largest Sloan-Kettering grants requests that had been put through in 1974 asked for $1,985,087 in the field of immunobiology and just over $2 million for molecular biology.

When these were approved by NCI, their funding was set at a total of just under $1.5 million, to which would be added the usual one third for overhead. If this sort of reduction, i.e., a 50 per cent cut, were applied to the institute's hoped-for core grant of $5 million, the budget situation might become untenable for Good.

Sloan-Kettering and its ebullient director were not the only ones to have exhibited an excess of optimism in 1974. Another sixty biomedical institutions around the nation were knocking at NCI's door that year with great expectations. Since Sloan-Kettering was the biggest cancer center, its expectations were also the largest. But this posed a problem for Rauscher. The NCI director made it clear that he was uneasy over the jealousy aroused in university biomedical circles by the size of the awards the East Sixty-eighth street facility might obtain under its formidably positioned chief.

Rauscher said, "We're talking about the issue of balance, which is the most complex and difficult, obviously, of all the issues we have. In regard to centers, I think it's a feel, and it's got to be a feel and it feels about right at the present time. I share the view of some that we may be in danger of putting too much money into centers. Some of my colleagues on the outside feel that when we recognize a center, they have a built-in advantage in getting competitive funds. I don't think that's true. Not yet anyway. We just have to assure people that every dollar that is spent has gone through the peer review process, be they grants, contracts, or what-have-you. I don't think we're doing this as well as we might at the present time. We have to be able to assure the Office of Management and Budget, the Congress, and the scientific community in general that individual scientists or groups of scientists in centers are in the same position as anyone else in competing for federal cancer dollars.

"We haven't done this communicating well. Even when I go to OMB right now when my budget reflects around $100 million for cancer centers, they have to understand that only $18 million of that is for core support and that the other $82 million is obtained by the centers' researchers in active competition for grants." Of course, Rauscher was speaking at a time when the biggest center on his list wasn't getting any core support. One wondered how the OMB was going to react to a cool $5 million in such support for Sloan-Kettering alone. As things stood at the beginning of fiscal 1975, the NCI was in good shape. It had $500 million from then President Nixon, another $23 million tacked on by the Congress, and $66 million in disimpounded funds. The cancer agency was then funding its grant requests at the rate of about 60 per cent.

Rauscher explained that fraction: "What you have to understand is that to fund even 50 per cent of new applications takes a whopping increase in money every year because once you approve a grant you are locked in to funding it for three years along with any increases that project may require. Consequently, if we don't get a lot of new money, we aren't able to fund new proposals coming in. I tend to agree with the Secretary [of Health, Education and Welfare, then Casper Weinberger] that if we keep on like this, we'll end up spending the whole national budget on cancer."

Some such thought must have been on the former Secretary's mind when his boss, Gerald Ford, finally got around to asking for some rescissions of expenditures in fiscal 1975. When the President's budget-chopping requests reached the Congress at the end of January, the rescission in NCI spending came in fourth after cuts in health services planning and development, agricultural conservation programs, and Air Force jet procurement. Congress was asked to approve spending $568.6 million for cancer, about $20 million less than in fiscal 1974 and $123 million less than the previous Congress had authorized.

A few days before the President offered another reminder to scientists of the impermanence of executive commitments to research, I sat in the lavishly appointed office of Benno Schmidt asking him what he had been telling the President about cancer spending. It had become obvious that some trimming of the cancer program was in the wind. Schmidt, from the offices of J. H. Whitney & Company high above Manhattan's Fifth Avenue, held the chairmanship of the President's advisory panel on cancer until the end of the following month, a post in the triumvirate he had held since Mr. Nixon appointed him early in 1972.

He was also a close enough friend of President Ford to have called the latter "Jerry" before his accession to the White House.

The Texas financier speaks slowly with a basso drawl that somehow doubles the weight of his words. He said first that he had not recently communicated with the President except in writing: "My own impression is that the President has a genuine and real interest in the cancer program but that, understandably, he has been so preoccupied with other things since he took office that he has not really had time or an opportunity to give the program the amount of personal time, personal attention, and personal support that I'm hopeful he'll give it when things clear away a little bit. [Things haven't.] Obviously his primary concerns are economics and energy." While Schmidt admitted to having corresponded with the White House about the major health posts then vacant—the under-secretary for health and the director of NIH—he made it clear that he was not nagging the President about NCI. He also made it clear that a rescission request of the kind that surfaced seventy-two hours later would not surprise him.

Reminiscing about the days when he headed the original Senate-appointed task force to look into what should be done to speed the conquest of cancer, Schmidt recalled, "As minority leader, President Ford arranged a luncheon for me with the leaders in the House of Representatives because I wanted to be sure that what we decided was called for wouldn't be approved by the Senate only to run into a brick wall in the House. It was a very good and reassuring lunch. Because of that, President Ford was sort of in at the beginning as far as the Cancer Act was concerned. He was always a strong supporter of the act and always available for all the help he could give me in the days when the act was pending. When he was Vice-President, he and I happened to be together on and off for a couple of days on one occasion, and we had occasion to talk about the cancer program in general, and he suggested the next time I was in Washington we set up a date and talk about it a little more." By that next time, however, Gerald Ford was President.

"Then," Schmidt rumbled, "I saw the President briefly on the afternoon when Mrs. Ford went to the hospital for her operation and he asked me how the cancer effort was going. I don't have any question that the President, in principle, is behind the best cancer effort that we're capable of. He is also behind a good medical research program. But right now that cuts across the recommendations he's getting from some of his staff about reducing federal expenditures in every area where it's possible to reduce them."

Then, going on to a prediction that rescission proposals would hit biomedical research along with other programs, Schmidt observed, "I understand that he can't make exceptions of everything that he's friendly toward or friendly disposed toward if we're gonna tighten our belt."

Schmidt's ensuing words then took on an almost elegiac quality as, paradoxically, the rhythm of his speech accelerated. "I don't happen to agree about medical research cutbacks. I wouldn't cut the NIH dollars. I have so advised the President in writing and have made what I consider to be the appropriate arguments as strongly as I can. I'm assured that those have had his personal attention and that he has quite a lot of sympathy for the arguments but that, dealing with the economic problems, he did not feel that he could make an exception and let the cancer budget stand where the Congress had put it." In short, Benno Schmidt had been reliably informed that, with appropriate regrets, the ax had once again been taken from the Executive rack for one of the larger, expendable lambs.

Even without a slash in the NCI budget, Schmidt conceded, Sloan-Kettering was in for a couple of very difficult years. There was, however, no hint in his replies to questions that the board of trustees of the institute (on which he sits with considerable weight as vice-chairman of Memorial Sloan-Kettering Cancer Center) would deviate from its decision to support Robert Good in his resetting of the research compass on Sixty-eighth Street. However, the J. H. Whitney executive had addressed himself to the center's $6.7 million deficit in a talk he gave there in December 1974. The deficit, he had said, was offset by using cash reserves (i.e., selling stocks and bonds at their ten-year bottom on the market) and by using unrestricted bequests. But, he had warned, "we cannot continue to operate at this kind of deficit."

When it came to a discussion of what the nation could afford
in medical research, Schmidt turned easily to financial parlance.
"The facilities and the highly skilled and trained manpower
required for this job will not be there in the future if we allow
our support to lag now. We must not dissipate this intellectual
and organizational establishment. It is a national asset . . . that
would take years to replace."

And: "If any well-run business were spending one hundred
billion dollars per year on medical care, it would be spending at
least five per cent of that amount on research to reduce those
costs. . . . Often it is the unforeseen and unforseeable results
that provide the biggest payoff . . . these expenditures are not
inflationary. Their discontinuance may well be inflationary. . . .
the Federal expenditures in biomedical research are leverage
dollars. Hundreds of millions of dollars worth of institutional facilities built by our universities and other philanthropic institutions, and thousands of people whose salaries are paid by these
institutions are mobilized in the cause of biomedical research by
the relatively few federal dollars that are spent in stimulating
this activity."

Despite these persuasively rational exhortations against renewed budget chopping, Schmidt indicated to me that he could
accept $30 to $60 million under $691 million for NCI for 1975
though he felt even more than 691 could have been fruitfully
spent. (It would be unfair to the presidential adviser not to take
note of his complaints against manpower-training cuts and other
slices taken from NIH partly as a consequence of the cancer
push.)

Back in August of 1974, The Wall Street Journal had warned
scientists about their criticism of targeted research such as
had gained so many dollars for the National Cancer Institute as
"gravest heresy." "If the world of science wants to preserve the
character of its basic research, it will have to be more careful—
and more candid—in explaining itself to the bureaucrats and
politicians who pay the bills."

Precisely. The whole business had started when science began
to sell its spun-off bonuses as justification for its support. The
market for knowledge as knowledge had never been very re-

warding. It was, indeed, implicit promises by scientists—or would-be scientists—to the public, to foundations, to financiers, to the insatiable engines of government, that had ultimately thrown such a lurid glare on a couple of painted mice. There, at any rate, in early 1975, sat thousands of scientists and their technicians and their secretaries and their administrators waiting to see who would go broke in cancer and who would prosper.

There sat Robert Good fourteen stories above East Sixty-eighth Street hopefully predicting fiscal stability at Sloan-Kettering by 1976 or the year after, while a still hopeful public, along with Representative Flood and Senator Magnuson, watched their newspapers and television sets waiting for word of the mriacle.

William Summerlin was getting ready to pack up his Darien effects for a move to the South. He could, after all, still make a living as a skin specialist treating eczema and psoriasis even if his own story of an encounter with fame and research glory didn't find a publisher.

By mid-March 1975 the United States Congress had decided to spend all of the $691 million it had appropriated for the cancer program whether President Ford liked it or not. But by then the academic murmurs of complaint and the accusations that the whole program was a betrayal not only of science but of public expectations had grown louder and more insistent. Whether the Summerlin affair had played any major role in this amplification was impossible to determine. The debate was, however, beginning to rouse people who could cause far more trouble for Rauscher and his lieutenants at NCI than Gerald R. Ford, a President who seemed totally out of touch with the Congress from which he had been so abruptly snatched by his predecessor.

The new trouble came from the typewriter of Daniel Greenberg, Barbara Culliton's predecessor at *Science* as the chief gadfly of government science and medicine programs. Greenberg had left the magazine at the end of 1970 to found his own Washington-based newsletter called *Science and Government Report*. Prior to his departure, his pages in the news and comment section of *Science* had been avidly read by those who enjoyed seeing the scientific foibles and follies of Congress and the Nixon and Johnson administrations skewered, along with sundry idiocies of the bureaucrats who managed them. The latter, especially at the Atomic Energy Commission and the National Institutes of Health, must have welcomed Greenberg's departure. His new readership would now shrink to a fraction of what he reached at *Science*. He might snipe and carp at the new cancer program, but he would no longer be in a position to rouse any concerted protest among the influential people in American science nor would his popgun be much heard amid the clamor of politicians championing their cancer winner.

This was true until late in 1974 when Greenberg ran out of patience with what he saw as misleading propaganda the NCI and the cancer society were spreading in endless handouts to the electronic and print mass media. So he sat down and wrote an article about the emperor's deshabille for the *Columbia Journalism Review*. And before he wrote, he went back over the cancer survival statistics of the forties, fifties, and sixties so he could compare them with those of the good-news-about-cancer seventies. Reviewing these figures now for the readers of the organ of the Columbia University School of Journalism, among whom are many of the nation's better-known columnists and newscasters, Greenberg portrayed an emperor clad, at best, in socks and underdrawers.

When the NCI later issued its official announcement specifying progress made in survival trends for white cancer patients diagnosed between 1960 and 1961, the compilers of the statistical hand-out chose to ignore one of the three cancers responsible for most U.S. fatalities from the disease. While the cancer institute omitted colon cancer from its tables based on 230,502 patients from Connecticut, California, Massachusetts, and half a dozen university medical centers around the nation, it said that five-year survivals with breast cancer had increased from 60 per cent in the 1950s to 64 per cent in the late 1960s. NCI attributed this to catching smaller tumors earlier on. Similarly, the Bethesda statisticians were able to find a 7 per cent increase in five-year survivals for patients with Hodgkin's disease. Lung cancer was ignored in the text of the hand-out, but an accompanying table showed five-year survivals for the most common fatal tumor of men to have increased only from 7 to 8 per cent between the 1950s and the period 1965–69. The cancers in which NCI found detectable improvement included those of the prostate, testicle, kidney, bladder, brain, thyroid, and larynx and melanoma of the skin. The improvements in this group ranged from 9 per cent in the relatively benign prostate cancer down to five percentage points for brain tumors.

These were the sort of numbers that Greenberg said showed how little the public had gotten for so much money spent. Columnist Nicholas Von Hoffman read Greenberg's piece and decided the topic was ready for airing to his Washington *Post* readers, those of his syndicated column, and listeners to his point of view over the Columbia Broadcasting System radio network. His summary of Greenberg's charges in February of 1975 made it clear at the higher echelons in Bethesda that the cancer-dollar debate was on again and the three-year honeymoon over.

By the end of March the New York *Times* was using one of the worst political pejoratives its editorial writers could muster when the terms "cancer" and "pork barrel" were linked in the headline of a *Times* opinion piece. The substance of the essay concerned the rush of congressmen hastening to grab a cancer center for their districts, replacements for the military air bases and supply dumps and proving grounds of the more bellicose sixties. By this time, the number of projected cancer treatment and research centers had jumped from sixteen to thirty-eight.

The *Times* editorial came only two weeks after a day-long symposium at the Massachusetts Institute of Technology in Cambridge. Former presidential science adviser (under John F. Kennedy) and president of MIT Jerome Wiesner, introduced a panel of distinguished speakers on the problems of cancer. Three of the six were Nobel laureates. They had been convened to dedicate a new MIT biological sciences building for which funds had been contributed by the Seeley G. Mudd Foundation. The building houses the MIT Center for Cancer Research and a Cell Culture Center. But the renowned engineering school, as Wiesner made clear in his opening remarks, wasn't about to affiliate with a hospital or clinical center. In the Mudd Building

basic knowledge about viruses and cells and cancer and cardiovascular disease would be pursued with as much government
money as could be decently garnered, but without the trappings
of cobalt machines and million-dollar whole-body radiation
scanners. The basic research to be undertaken at MIT was not to
be tied with cancer-patient therapy along the lines of a Sloan-
Kettering Institute or an M. D. Anderson or a Roswell Park
tumor center.

Thus the two leaders of MIT cancer research, Nobelist and
virologist Dr. Salvador E. Luria, the director, and David Baltimore, Ph.D., enzymologist and molecular geneticist, did not
need to worry too much about whom they invited to discuss
the nation's cancer course setting since they had a foot in both
camps. Their research was, in large measure, being funded by
NCI, but they weren't some grubby little establishment in Kansas
or Kentucky or Nebraska putting up a front to bag some cancer
money, mainly for patient care with only a dollop of research
thrown in.

In Cambridge on that day early in March, two of the speakers
addressed themselves directly to the question that had been vexing some scientists since the budget of the National Institutes of
Health had been so tipped in favor of funding of cancer and
heart disease research in 1972. What should be the proper relationship, they asked, between funding basic research to turn up
new leads in cancer via new knowledge of how higher animal
cells behave as opposed to money funding studies of how better
to detect cancer and how to bring the optimum of today's therapeutic talent to most American cancer patients, a minority of
whom are now treated in existing centers?

One of the questioners was Nobel laureate James Watson,
professor of molecular biology at Harvard and director of the
famed Cold Spring Harbor Laboratory on Long Island's North
Shore. Watson, educated in Indiana and under Luria, has held
a professorship at Harvard for two decades since the DNA
elucidation at Cambridge University that brought him fame. He
still delights in attacking the Establishment when he thinks it is
wrong. As recorded earlier in this history, Watson is convinced
that the direction set for cancer control in 1972 is disastrously
muddled.

Watson's audience that day in Massachusetts was composed, it may be assumed, of numerous youthful scientists who will have to solve or aid in solving the myriad problems of how cells regulate each other, talk to each other, and change roles in ways that are constructive for or destructive of the organizations, i.e., bodies, they constitute. That young audience could be presumed to be knowledgeable about the stunningly perceptive new immunologic probes developed for such pursuits over the past decade as well as of the huge gaps in this body of knowledge.

As befitted a guest in the house, Watson began by complimenting his hosts. "What MIT has done is very sensible and wise. It has used the facts that more cancer money is available and that intelligent foundations exist, to create something new. You might say that any intelligent university would do the same, but, I fear MIT's course is unique. It is the only nonclinical American institution that has responded to the 'War on Cancer' in this grand way. But MIT must pay the penalty for acting more responsibly. It must carry a greater burden in seeing to it that fundamental cancer research is carried out in a sensible way over the next decades."

Then he turned his attention to the climate that produced our National Cancer Act. Said Harvard's Watson, "Starting in the 1940s with the Committee on Growth of the National Research Council there was the general consensus that if you were going to seriously study cancer, you had to generate more pure biology. That is, the science of biology was then not in a state where you could think sensibly about the cancer problem. So both the federal government through its various agencies and the American Cancer Society realized that they had to do something for pure, irrelevant science. The Cancer Society, for example, funded my first summer [1948] at Cold Spring Harbor studying bacterial viruses [phages] under Dr. Luria. It was all too clear that biology had to be nourished out of its predilection for descriptive analysis, and that this might be accomplished if you learned the key messages of the new physics and chemistry that had come out of university science departments in the 1920s and 1930s and started applying them to the major problems of experimental biology.

"Happily this revolution did occur and between 1945 and 1965 biology was transformed from a largely descriptive nature into a science with ample analytical powers. At the same time, the health lobbyists, whose enthusiasm had generated the initial flow of governmental and foundation cash, more and more began to think in terms of the human payoffs that soon should blossom forth. Here we must realize that twenty years [1945–65] in the average person's life is a long time. Moreover, it is only when you reach forty-five or so that you begin to have the ability to influence (lobby) the so-called older establishment. So after twenty years of influence you may be near sixty-five and realize that only a few more years may remain for you to see something happen out of your efforts. By 1970 we had reached that stage in the lives of our key cancer lobbyists, and since it was universally agreed that biology had come of age, it seemed almost natural, if not God ordained to them, that the new biology should bring a halt to the horrors of cancer.

"At the same time, those of us who had participated in the birth of the new biology, largely by doing experiments on the most simple cells, the bacteria and their viruses, the phages, began to realize that now was the time to move onto the world of the much more complicated cells of higher animals. With luck, we might begin to understand the essence of embryological development as well as possibly coming to grips with the essence of cancer cells. But we worried that we might not have enough money, for no matter how we might proceed, the need for much more money, seemed unavoidable. And so, as the 1970s broke, there existed two independent pushes for lots of new cancer money. To be sure, they had two very different immediate goals, one to cure cancer, the other to understand it. In any case, our country was thought to be coming out of its greatest national debacle and both the clinicians and the pure scientists thought there should be money saved from Vietnam that could be used for cancer research."

During the original Yarborough hearings and those that later followed to draft precise legislation, Watson recalled that he and several colleagues had testified that further study of the so-called cancer viruses was likely to be the most direct way to get at the genetic basis of cancer. Though he admitted his advice was parochial since he himself would use some of this cancer virus money, he said he felt sure that such money, if properly spent, could not fail to pay off eventually by telling us exactly the enzymatic basis by which a cell becomes cancerous. He went on to say that "other witnesses, many more in number, testified that at long last we are beginning to cure by chemicals some forms of disseminated cancer (e.g., chorocarcinoma) that we couldn't cure before. Give us the money to set up additional large cancer centers like the Memorial Sloan-Kettering complex, and over the next decade we can cure even more cancers either by better use of anti-cancer drugs or through new immunological procedures. Though both types of testimony helped insure the eventual passage of the conquest of cancer legislation, there is no doubt that it was the latter testimony about possible cures over the next decade—'a billion a year for ten years will do the job'—that created the climate for its unanimous passage and immediate funding. It is the lobby which says we may have real results in five to ten years that carries the day. Talk about longer intervals and everyone gets bored, at least those over fifty which includes almost all of our Congressmen.

"In fact, I used to ask for money for our Cold Spring Harbor Lab on that schedule. Give us the money to get further inside the animal cell and in five to ten years we will begin to understand and may start to cure more cancer. But now, after seven years, I find it hard to throw out the same old message. For the more we learn about normal higher cells and their cancerous equivalents, the more staggering the task I realize we have cut out for ourselves. We may easily have twenty-five to fifty years ahead of us as pure scientists before we can precisely say, for example, why a cell has become leukemic. This does not mean nothing of consequence will happen sooner. In fact, the science of cancer goes increasingly well, and every new year, if not month, brings forth something we now momentarily think to be a fundamental lead. But we must be very careful not to confuse our day-by-day intellectual thrills with a thorough understanding of the nature of cancer. To do so is cheating, and while the rewards for perpetual enthusiastic optimism may be piles of soft money, the long-term result has to be loss of intellectual integrity. Nonetheless, when I say my long-term goal is merely to understand cancer, not to cure it, I fear that not only will I be deemed socially irresponsible, but that I will find it increasingly hard to get money for a goal which does not directly aim to help the immediate sick or those who soon will be so."

Then Watson inquired what had been done with the doubling of U.S. cancer funds, even allowing for inflation, that had occurred since passage of the cancer legislation. To start, he characterized its over-all plan, "the National Cancer Plan," as largely a public relations effort. Initially conceived as the flow chart for a Polaris missile-type approach to cancer, it grew out of a number of meetings of cancer experts at Airlie House, a conference center in Virginia. Though the conferences produced evidence of large numbers of possible leads into cancer, Watson found the final massively heavy plan a total sham which carefully took care not to distinguish between the respective merits of the so-called hot leads. "Nowhere can you find directions to spend more here and less there. So at best it is a catalogue of wishful thinking to which the director of the NCI can point in front of Congress and say 'Yes, we know where we are going.' But during my two years experience on the National Cancer Advisory Board it never had any impact on anyone and in general the doubling in total funds has merely allowed most pre-existing progress to become twice as large, thereby not again coming to grips with a real set of priorities.

"In fact, the only two new directions taken by the NCI both evolved out of the direct dictates of the 1971 cancer legislation. The first was an expansion of the pre-existing center program in the direction of the creation of new comprehensive cancer centers. The models used to justify this expansion were the Memorial Sloan-Kettering complex, the newly created Dana complex in Boston, Rosewell Park in Buffalo, and the M. D. Anderson complex in Houston. Twelve new complete centers were to be created to bring the total number to sixteen. As such, they were to be concerned with all aspects of the cancer problem, both clinical and nonclinical and so to cover everything from the cause of cancer to the rehabilitation of patients who have been treated for cancer.

"Unfortunately, from the very start, the politics of where these new centers should be located has occupied much more attention than whether their concept really makes that much sense. While

clearly no one is against better cancer treatment, it does not
necessarily follow that putting the so-called pure scientist under
the same organizational framework as the cancer clinician will
make them collaborate. In fact, it might be wiser to place the
best of our scientists working on cancer next to the best of
our graduate students, say, at Caltech rather than close to the
patient at a Los Angeles cancer hospital. But for better or worse
—and I fear much the worse—the 1971 cancer legislation gave
heavy legitimatization to the concept of the massive cancer
centers. This, despite the fact that the pre-existing past history
of our comprehensive centers, gives us no reason to believe they
would be the best setting for research programs that could be
the most difficult that biologists have yet tried to pull off.

"But we did not talk about this during meetings of the Cancer
Board, only considering, say, whether Denver or Seattle made
more sense as a location for a center. To be sure, in a democracy
there is every reason to fight for the idea of rapidly making
medical care equal in all geographical regions. But as in the
war on poverty, the question must be either whether we had
chosen achievable short-term objectives. It is very hard to create
anything of excellence in a short time, particularly massive
cancer centers, when there is anything but an oversupply of
doctors expert in chemotherapy or the still more elusive immunotherapy. No matter how hard you try, you can't pull qualified specialists out of a hat. If you don't have deep clinical
expertise and imagination, your potential center in Boise, Idaho,
for example, will give no better treatment than that already
provided by its general hospital.

"Nonetheless, from the very start the concept of comprehensive centers was a sacred cow and the NCI, responding to the
wishes of a large majority of the Cancer Board, set out to bring
them into existence as quickly as possible. Essentially, the lobbying that produced this climate stated that many more lives
could be saved if we set up the centers and so being against
them was like arguing against motherhood. But I have never
heard any good estimate on how many lives could be saved,
and so it may be impossible to decide whether they work any
better than the best of our local hospitals. Of course, it would
be a very different matter if now we had the means to cure the

disseminated form of any major cancer (e.g., colon or breast). If that were the case, then those potentially very expensive centers would clearly make sense. But I fear we don't, and I suspect that we may be pushing a concept that only can be really successful if completely new forms of treatment emerge. But as of this moment, the hot leads are all exceedingly border-line. In any case, I fear, that it will be impossible to shut down a comprehensive cancer center even if, at best, it is only mar-ginally more effective than other local hospitals. It will be even more difficult than trying to close down an antiquated VA hos-pital.

"To be sure, doubts were occasionally raised, and I recall at several meetings of the National Cancer Board that Benno Schmidt said we should not go beyond the originally asked for sixteen centers. But by now thirty appear to be the target, and I will be surprised if less than forty exist a decade from now. For it will be difficult, if not impossible, to withhold from a high population center the possession of a highly touted 'comprehen-sive cancer center,' even though there may be no statistical yard-stick by which their supposed superiority over that of our best noncancer hospital centers can be proved.

"Such sentimental decisions, however, may become increas-ingly large albatrosses in the aftermaths of the Vietnamese de-bacle and our oil-induced current recession. When the dollars for cancer research cease to grow, will we find that we have created a significant number of first-rate centers for cancer re-search like the one MIT has just founded, or will we have committed all too much of our money for a hollow façade that can't be torn down? Alas, if we only ask this question of the doctors in charge of the comprehensive clinical centers, we can expect reports of glowing progress. So it will pay, painful as it may be, to find ways of having such judgments made by people whose future careers are not tightly bound to their con-tinued funding.

"The second congressionally mandated cancer program was that of Cancer Control. This was to be a funding device to bring better diagnosis and treatment to the average victim. Ini-tially funded for only twenty-five million dollars, this program will soon grow to some one hundred million dollars, and could easily consume vastly greater sums if, happily, it can work. But early detection is tricky to bring off and except for the Pap test is not easily achieved. Now the main new thrust of the control program goes toward breast cancer, a most obvious goal considering its steady pernicious rise and the relatively young age at which it can strike. But it is far from clear whether over a long-term interval you can achieve large-scale early detection without turning American women into hopeless nervous wrecks. And the same psychological facts of life argue against the early detection of most other major cancers.

"But since Cancer Control so directly brings the national cancer program to the general public, it seems bound to grow and very easily could consume a third, if not more, of the total NCI budget. Here we should be very clear that the essence of the program is not research but immediate help to our nation's people. So unless we have some way of accurately judging its success, it could acquire a momentum that could directly depress the money that goes toward understanding, if not preventing, the major cancers. Considering the vast sums probably necessary if very early detection is ever to be achieved on a national scale, we may find that it makes most sense to spend much of this money to see that known environmental carcinogens are kept away from the American public. But such a goal will bring the NCI into direct conflict with very powerful industrial lobbies, and at least when I was on the Board there was a noted reluctance for the NCI to take on any regulatory role.

"On the more positive side, the new cancer money has permitted about every form of cancer research to get more money. Viral oncology, chemical carcinogenesis, the biology of the cancer cell, as well as programs for the development of new drugs, are all financially much better off. But here we should note that most of this new money has gone to institutions and companies already engaged in large scale cancer research before the passage of the new cancer legislation. The only major exception is the center we are here today dedicating. So essentially, we are placing most of our faith, that is, money, in the intellectual traditions of the cancer research world that existed prior to the Act. At the same time the nonclinical, academically based biological community, such as the part of Harvard I come from, has gotten much poorer in an absolute sense. Yet it has been this academic nonclinical world which has largely been responsible for the amazing development of the new biology of the past twenty-five years. So we may be witnessing a transference of power [money] from the research-oriented universities that have made American biology as it now exists, to a new power base whose past existence was derived from its willingness to work on cancer at a time when most scientists thought it to be an intellectual graveyard.

"Here we must not solely fault the National Cancer Institute and its advisers. Instead, much blame must also fall on our leading pure science institutions for not realizing that what they are now doing may in the long term contribute more to a cure for a major cancer than any of the so-called relevant research now done in the official cancer centers. So instead of initiating large-scale programs in animal cell biology and asking for commensurate construction funds to house such activities, they have let the major expansion made possible by the conquest of cancer legislation fall to those institutions that already had development [fund raising] offices geared toward cancer and who at the first hint of piles of new money assembled the architects to draw up plans for the new comprehensive centers. So all too often the NCI has had to place their money with institutions of doubtful intellectual tradition and created still others in intellectual environments not known to foster bold science.

"It would be far better to be slow in the starting of new cancer research institutes than staff them with scientists not at home with the best of contemporary biology. For unless we wish to place all our faith in pure luck, we must realize that high-quality cancer research is likely to be much more difficult to pull off than most other forms of biology. We must never forget that we are largely in it not because it is the next obvious objective on an intellectual basis, but because of a desire to alleviate a major source of human suffering. Now even though the quality of the best of cancer research is at least on a par with the best of modern biology, we must again accept the fact that all too many of the challenging problems in cancer are at best marginally attackable with today's methodologies. So a brighter intellectual sparkle may be required for successful cancer research than for, say, the current challenges of microbial molecular genetics. Yet I would be less than honest if I said that I thought the average quality of the American scientist doing cancer research is rapidly going up. At this moment I fear it is at best holding its own because we have chosen to place most of the new efforts in institutions who never had much success in attracting the very best.

"So we must not be surprised that for the first time visible attacks on the national cancer program are beginning to appear. The trouble now in the cancer clinic is not that plausible new approaches are being overlooked in favor of past sterility. It is, as I emphasized earlier, that we may not have even one really hot clinical lead that has a good chance to lead somewhere soon with a major cancer. So we must be much more careful than we have in the past as to what we allow our lobbyist friends to claim for us. We must not passively sit and listen to people who through overoptimism or premature senility promise things that are very unlikely to happen soon. We have watched too much of this over the past few years. We should do the science we are trained for and not hold the carrot too close. We have to sell ourselves, in short, for what we really are, and not for our dreams that the knowledge we now obtain can be immediately applied against some terrible form of cancer.

"But if we respond to the fear of less cancer money for next year by flashing out even shakier new leads, say, in tumor immunology, to mask the fact that we still have not made the big breakthrough, we have nowhere to go but down. Eventually the general public will come to regard the scientific community as it does governmental press officers. Nevertheless, I fear that as more attacks on the war on cancer materialize, the NCI may feel it can only defend itself well by asking for still more money. The easiest thing to do when you don't know what to do is to ask for more cash. So we must expect that they will be greatly tempted to ask for still more money for still more comprehensive cancer centers and still more cancer control, blaming the lack of clinical progress not on lack of real new ideas or clinical procedures but on the unavailability of money to carry out achievable objectives.

"The best thing I think our country can now do in the war against cancer is create just one more institute of high quality cancer research equivalent to what MIT has started here today. That will do more than all the official hoopla we now receive through the daily mail and the press."

Another speaker that March day in Cambridge had another suggestion relating to the proportion of money that should be spent on applied or relevant cancer research as against basic biological inquiries on molecular genetics, cell surface interactions, viruses, enzymes and other matters. Dr. Michael G. P. Stoker spoke not in the hurried gasps of Watson, but in the measured and sonorous tones of an English don. He is director of the Imperial Cancer Research Fund Laboratories in London, an institution which raises its own funds through public appeals and private grants but is barred from receiving any money from Her Majesty's government.

Stoker said, "It's generally agreed that a simple causal chain between fundamental research and the useful application of it is very rare. . . . Professor Harry Johnson [of organic chemistry at the University of California] has the concept of basic research contributing to a pool in which the applied scientist fishes. The result is a lack of temporal correlation between the acquisition of the elements of knowledge that go into the pool and their subsequent appearance in useful application. My idea is that some mechanism should be found by which cancer funds can be used for the maintenance and expansion of this pool of general knowledge. What I'm proposing, in effect, is a sort of levy or tax on cancer money to help pay for its dependence in research on strategic biology."

Stoker was quick to see the trouble with his own scheme, the precise line to be drawn in a rather murky area where biology for the sake of knowledge becomes biology for the sake of attacking cancer. But the British scientist said he felt such a point on the gradient, as he termed it, could be located.

Now, of course, Frank Rauscher and those who head the cancer program in the United States could answer Stoker with considerable justification that they *do* fund basic biological research endeavors, but despite the Briton's confidence that a time could be drawn, any attempt by the NCI to claim that certain

grants fund strategic or basic research would produce a donny-
brook in science that would make the furor about the Zinder
Committee report look like a game of chess.

When word of Watson's charges reached Rauscher, his reply
was simple. He insisted that progress had been made against cancer of high incidence and mortality. He said, "It will be 1978 and
later before we know, based on five-year survival rates, just how
successful our efforts in the past two years have been. I don't
know of a single responsible scientist who ever promised Congress
we were going to find some magic bullet overnight."

When a writer recently asked Memorial Sloan-Kettering's president, Dr. Thomas, the biology-watcher, for his views on progress against cancer, he replied, "We still do not understand
the mechanism of this disease with sufficient authority. And it is
my claim that when we do have this kind of profound understanding of the mechanisms, we will then be able to take the appropriate measures to think our way around the disease." Thomas
is not only cautious in his utterances, but some might even find
him about as negative as Watson. Later in the same interview
he said, "I am quite prepared for the eventuality that the cause
of cancer is something no one has yet thought of. In fact, I
would not be surprised to learn that we are all wrong at the
present time. This has happened before in science, and, while I
wouldn't say that I expect it to go that way, I think the odds are
fairly good that we will be surprised."

Of course, Watson's reply to that would be that our chances of
being surprised depend in good measure on how strategically the
net is spread. He is partly wrong, I believe, in choosing the new
network of cancer centers as the central target for his attack.
If one has worked around a cancer center, the moans of expert
surgeons, radiologists, and chemotherapists are frequently heard.
The latex-gloved handwringing at Memorial and Rosewell Park
and M. D. Anderson at Cedars Sinai and Mount Sinai, at
Columbia Presbyterian and Methodist hospitals is occasioned
by the botched patients the medical center physicians see after
a local general surgeon or other practitioner has fooled around
with the seriously stricken cancer patient, giving him a harm-
less and totally ineffective dose of radiation or drugs or cutting
away part of the cancer, sewing the patient back up and telling

him he is fine. Obviously, if there are more centers of clinical
expertise in cancer, and obviously if the public hears about such
places, there will be less need for oncologists at the existing
medical centers to treat—or try to treat—patients who had a
chance and missed it in inept hands.

But when Watson wonders whether there is enough research
talent to go around, he is obviously on firm ground. The stam-
pede for government money has been producing a game of
musical chairs—sometimes endowed and sometimes not—in the
nation's major medical centers that serves mainly to run up the
salary bills. Good's arrival in New York with his phalanx of fifty
was by no means unique except, perhaps, in the size of his en-
tourage. Instead of budgeting like prudent people on fixed in-
comes, those who run the centers look with covetous eyes on the
superstar who is resident elsewhere. Now such a man or woman
is wooed with ardor and promises—expensive promises. The
medical centers' budgets are thrown away. Laboratories are
built or remodeled. Technicians are hired, expensive devices are
bought. All this is done in the expectation of NIH funding to
come. It is as if some sensible householders, hearing that rich
Uncle Harry has the flu, promptly ankle down to the nearest
Cadillac dealer to trade in the Pinto wagon. This is the sort of
hysteria that worries Watson, and no matter that Rauscher is
technically correct in assaying promises to Congress by scientists
—there are hundreds of foundation directors and wealthy individuals who are being cajoled with baseless cancer promises and
there are plenty of congressmen, like Daniel Flood, who have
somehow been led to expect the hallelujah next week.

In medicine, a sign of a disease, such as an elevated temperature, is termed a "symptom." The totality of its signs is called a
"syndrome." The pressure that William Summerlin felt when he
came to New York, together with the glow of the easily won
fame and publicity, the temptation that Robert Good felt not to
watch too closely while his protégé speeded up the pace of transplantation progress, and Memorial Sloan-Kettering's reward to
Summerlin of $40,000 to just go away quietly after he was caught
—these may be accounted a syndrome of a disease that this
writer believes Watson has accurately diagnosed.

EPILOGUE

The Responsibility of the Media

VETERINARIANS WERE yipping and caterwauling like their patients on the table when word got out in 1969 that cats with lymphosarcoma, the feline version of human leukemia, harbored a virus that was capable of producing tumors in newborn kittens, puppies, rabbits, and marmosets.

In 1970 public health doctors from the New York State Department of Health said they had evidence that Hodgkin's disease, a lymphatic cancer, *could* be transmitted between persons who were in close contact.

In 1971 Dr. Sol Spiegelman and Dr. Jeffrey Schlom of the Columbia Presbyterian Medical Center in New York City revealed indirect evidence for the presence of an RNA virus closely related to one that causes mammary tumors in mice in the breast tissue and milk of women with breast cancer. Dr. Dan Moore of the Institute for Medical Research in Camden, New Jersey, had earlier reported detecting a so-called "B-virus" in the milk of Parsee women in India, who were noted for their susceptibility to breast cancer, and in the milk of American women with a family history of that form of carcinoma. Dr. Spiegelman said: "If it were my sister [that is, a woman with a strong family history], I would advise her not to nurse."

The bovine tuberculosis vaccine BCG that had cleared up a few surface nodules of human malignant melanoma and cured some guinea pigs of a similar cancer was rashly touted as a "most significant breakthrough" by Dr. Michael Hanna, a distinguished scientist at the Oak Ridge National Laboratory, closely associated with the NCI, in the fall of 1972. That year, too, F. Kingsley Sanders, Ph.D., and Magdalena Eisinger, D.V.M., of the Sloan-Kettering Institute suggested they might have isolated a herpes virus that was associated with Hodgkin's disease.

In 1973 came Dr. Albert Sabin's herpes virus pronouncement, and in 1974, NCI's Frank Rauscher told the United Press International one Sunday that "dramatic new findings by a breast cancer task force indicate the traditional type of radical surgery undergone by First Lady Betty Ford offers no advantages over a less mutilating technique."

Were these various pronouncements right or wrong? In most cases the final answers are still not available. Five years after the report on feline lymphosarcoma it has been established that cats can transmit this form of cancer among their own species, but no instance of spread to humans has yet been documented. Four years after the suggestion that Hodgkin's disease is transmissible, more epidemiologic data has been gathered by Dr. Nicholas Vianna and his colleagues, but NCI doesn't believe it. Three years after Spiegelman said that women with a strong history of breast cancer shouldn't breast-feed their babies, there is no new evidence that the B-viruses are transmissible in human milk, though there is added proof that the method used for detecting them is a sound one.

We live in a thicket of instant communication. Scientists egged on by their hungry institutions not only compete for grant money but for the Nobel prize, as James Watson so accurately related. In addition, the subject of cancer seems to bring out latent indiscretion in many scientists, perhaps because with the Cancer Act of 1971 there is so much money available for research. Compared with some of the agonizing (to cancer patients and their friends and relatives) misinformation that has been circulated by the nation's wire services, magazines, television and radio stations, and newspapers in the years since the Cancer Act was passed, Good's espousal of Dr. Summerlin's transplant "breakthrough" sometimes appears almost pallidly inconsequential.

When scientists who would not think of painting a mouse, doctoring a notebook, or otherwise touching up their data speak to the press, there is almost always some inexperienced wire-service reporter listening. Once the story makes the national and so-called "radio" wire, there are not usually any further strainers between it and the public. The handful of radio and television stations that employ science or medical specialists wouldn't think of calling them up at home to clear an item promising progress against cancer that the Associated Press, United Press International, or Reuters had put on the wire. The news editors assume it has been passed by a science man at the news desk of the hired service. Out goes the "breakthrough" dispatch to every home and auto in the nation. Next day the scientist explains that he was misquoted or didn't have time to voice appropriate reservations. Then a correction or amplification runs over the wire, but nobody out there on the receiving end pays any attention.

Does public excitement over stories that are carefully told and reported gain funding for scientists or for their institutions? The answer must be a guarded "probably." Money does come in from private contributors thanks to such stories, and the big foundations and corporate givers often ask an institution's fund raiser, "Well, what have you done over there lately?" If they have seen a headline about one of the institution's scientists in their local newspaper or heard something on television or on the radio recently, they are less likely to be picky and more inclined to give the money. The opposite effect, caused by jealousy, may sometimes be seen at NCI, however, where a scientist's sudden fame inspires a little off-the-record blood-letting by colleagues who see a chance to profit by calling him "unprofessional" or a "publicity hound."

Two of the items mentioned earlier in this chapter require explanation if readers are not going to run for the nearest doctor or hospital every time they read a headline or hear a bulletin. I've chosen one from the surgical area and one dealing with cancer immunotherapy. In both, more attention to telling the "how" of the story and a little more attention to the background would have enormously benefited reader understanding and prevented unnecessary grief. In both, there was the chance for editors to have reined in their reporters by seeking some expert advice at the main news bureau. In neither case was this done.

The news stories about needless radical mastectomy ran, coincidentally, just a day or so after President Ford's wife had undergone one in 1974. Controversy had been raging for ten years and longer over the merits of surgery in which only the cancerous lump in the breast is removed, the cutting off of the entire affected breast, and the latter operation plus excision of the underlying chest muscles and the chain of about thirty lymph nodes that run down under the armpit and drain the breast on that side—the first adjacent tissues to be exposed to tumor cells straying from their primary site. The third operation is the one known as "radical," which in surgical terms means extensive in scope, not innovative.

The stories that ran in the newspapers and on television and radio said that the controversy had been settled by a large NCI joint study in which many surgeons and hospitals had been participating since 1971. According to the news articles and bulletins, the study said the radical operation had not been proved superior to simple breast removal. This led many women who had suffered the additional discomfort and disability of the radical operation to wonder why their doctors had talked them into it or insisted upon it.

What the news stories did not mention was that the evaluation had to be a preliminary one on the basis of its own avowed time scale. Meticulous cancer researchers in the clinical arena avoid retrospective studies. No matter how carefully the doctors and biostatisticians examine records of previous operations, they cannot be certain that there wasn't bias in the selection of the patients for the procedures to be compared or that there weren't slight but important differences in how the patients were treated.

In a prospective study, on the other hand, the participating doctors—in this instance, breast surgeons—can get together and agree on rigid rules of patient selection, the stage of the disease at operation—tiny, large, metastasized, etc.—and the extent of the surgery and the terms of the aftercare. All well and good. The only trouble with the results announced by the NCI was that data from only three years of the *prospective* study were available. To give the radical mastectomy surgeons their due, they have based their argument on what they see as enhanced five-, ten-, and fifteen-year survivals. They regard a two-year survival as meaningless since so many women now have breast lumps detected early and operated on early.

But the news media at first were so busy getting comments from Mrs. Ford's surgeon that they neglected to inform their audience of an extremely important facet of the big government survey.

United Press Washington reporter Edward Delong, for example, interviewed Rauscher the day before the results of the NCI breast cancer study were officially released. His article, filed on September 29, 1974, began: "Dramatic new findings by a breast cancer task force indicate the traditional type of radical surgery undergone by Betty Ford offers no advantages over a less mutilating technique, the head of the National Cancer Institute said Sunday." In his third paragraph, Delong mentioned in passing that the NCI study had been started in 1971, but Delong did not use the word "preliminary" in his story, whether because Rauscher neglected to emphasize the brevity of the study or because Delong, a technology reporter, didn't think the length of the study was important. When the UPI's chief science writer wrote a second story out of the meeting the following day, he noted in his sixth paragraph that the findings reported were "preliminary." But the New York *Times,* which had carried the original story in its late city edition, had to ask one of their own science reporters, Jane Brody, to clarify the status of the radical mastectomy a few days later. And she did.

The second incident, in which editors and broadcasters threw away their caution and broke out their "cancer breakthrough" lead paragraphs, began innocuously enough in September 1972 with an announcement from the NCI of a major conference that would pull together what was then known about the use of BCG vaccine in the immunologic attack on tumors. It was a routine press release running about four pages and listing the participants in the forthcoming meeting. Thinking, however, to give the uninitiated some background on the potential of this new form of treatment, government public information officers tacked onto the end of the announcement a description of some recent work in which melanoma induced in guinea pigs had melted away when the animals were injected with BCG. The laboratory work, the release said, had been done by three respected NCI investigators whose names and locations were given. One of the three, Dr. Hanna, performed his research at Oak Ridge, Tennessee, in a laboratory normally devoted to investigating cancer causation.

One of the rules of publicity handouts dictates that one should always mail to the home-town papers and wire services. The Associated Press and United Press International bureaus that cover the Oak Ridge National Laboratory from day to day are located in Knoxville. The publicity arm of the NCI, therefore, mailed the BCG conference announcement to the wire service bureaus in Knoxville because of Hanna's involvement. Knoxville UPI plowed through the announcement and read about the guinea pigs, their melanoma, and their BCG treatment.

Knoxville UPI then filed a cancer story to its main office, the Atlanta bureau. Atlanta found the Knoxville file a little conservative and dull. The Atlanta bureau is in charge of all southern region news and its manager can handle a story any way he wants. In this case, he turned it over to a reporter in the Nashville UPI bureau for a little improvement. She called Dr. Hanna and he said some things he probably shouldn't have said about

BCG. By this time it was Friday, September 22. The Nashville reporter then filed the revised story to Atlanta. Atlanta liked it and sent it along to UPI headquarters in New York.

The United Press International does not believe in specialists. Its credo is that any newsman worthy of the name can cover anything. UPI had had to assign a new science writer to their New York office in the 1950s. In line with their philosophy of scientifically naïve news coverage, the UPI brass chose their music critic for this job. As it turned out, it was a happy choice. The late Delos Smith, the former music critic, turned to with a will, combing the pages of *The British Medical Journal, The Lancet, The New England Journal of Medicine,* and other medical periodicals and covering the field admirably considering that he had no help and scarcely any travel budget. In September 1972, however, Smith was confined to his New York apartment. Lung cancer and the radiation and drugs given him in a futile attempt to save his life had weakened his bones, and one day, when struggling to pull on his rubbers, he had broken his hip.

The UPI reporters had no one to check their story with, nobody to tell them that reports on BCG from several cancer centers had already indicated some therapeutic effects against melanoma confined to the skin and also some life-threatening side reactions, and offered the possibilities discussed in an earlier chapter. Once the "breakthrough" story from Oak Ridge's Dr. Hanna was on its way to New York and to the world, there was a last chance to save the day by calling Smith. But the wire service editors in Manhattan didn't take it.

At about six o'clock that Friday night, September 22, Barbara Yuncker of the New York *Post* was driving to her country house north of New York when her car radio blared the news of a new cancer drug called BCG that was accomplishing wonders. As soon as she got to the next gasoline station on the Taconic State Parkway, reporter Yuncker went to the phone booth and put in a call to the *Post*. She intended to warn her editors against the story she had just heard, a story she rightly assumed was being disseminated by one or both wire services. In two tries, owing to the vagaries of the telephone system, she was unable to reach her newspaper and gave up, figuring her editors would call her anyway before they put such an article in the weekend *Post*. She was wrong.

Editors at the Associated Press over in Rockefeller Center also heard the news. They had been scooped. Available to them were five competent science writers, two in New York and one each in Washington, Houston, and Los Angeles. None were called. Instead, a bureau man from Knoxville was dispatched to catch up with Hanna and the big cancer story.

At 11:59 the most widely disseminated news service in the world (with the possible exception of British Reuters) told the world: "Scientists at Oak Ridge National Laboratory say they have discovered a cancer treatment that is the 'most significant breakthrough in reduction of tumors by immunology' to date. Dr. Michael Hanna, Jr., said Friday that injection of the chemical, BCG, into tumors grown in laboratory animals has resulted in 100 per cent elimination of metastasis, the medical term for the spread of cancer cells to other sites in the body. But he cautioned that BCG treatment could not yet be called a 'cure' for all cancers that affect human beings . . ."

The story went on for four more paragraphs, concluding, "Hanna said he hoped the treatment would soon be tested on a larger number of cancer sufferers. 'It's difficult to say when it could become a standard treatment,' he said."

Thanks to the naïvete of a scientist and to the thoughtless hunger of a handful of editors for a cancer scoop, telephones began ringing Saturday morning at every cancer hospital in the country, at Bethesda, and at Oak Ridge. They went on ringing for days. The callers were relatives of doomed cancer victims begging for some of the magic the wire service genies had summoned.

By Saturday afternoon, the Associated Press, at least, was trying to stuff the genie back in the bottle. Washington reporter Martha Cole talked with Hanna's co-author, Dr. Herbert J. Rapp of the NCI and at 4 P.M. the AP carried a dispatch on its wires that made clear that BCG was in no sense ready for widespread testing against cancer. But the big news was out and there are few editors left in city rooms late on Saturday afternoon. The New York *Post* and dozens of other major dailies around the country had played the story big. Those like the New York *Times*, whose editors consulted their science writers, ignored it.

By Tuesday, September 26, when the flap over BCG still hadn't died down, the AP editors thought they had better try another clarification. Now one of their science reporters, Brian Sullivan, was belatedly assigned to the task. He did the best he could. The result sent over the wire on Wednesday was more of an apology than a news item: "Scientists at the Oak Ridge National Laboratory say they regret that a misunderstanding over a cancer research report last weekend led to a widespread but false belief that there had been a major advance toward a treatment for cancer." Sullivan's story also reported that Oak Ridge had received hundreds of calls from across the United States and from other nations including Japan, Britain, Argentina, and Australia. Hanna was quoted as saying, "I feel apologetic to the people who telephoned me and certainly to the outsiders who sought me out at the laboratory."

As for the UPI, a few months later I had occasion to write to the wire service's editor-in-chief, H. L. Stevenson, about the BCG fiasco. He shot back, "I've carefully examined the copy we filed, the statements made by the Tennessee doctor involved and I am convinced the fault does not lie with us." Stevenson has never had to take any telephone calls in a cancer hospital. In his view, apparently, if his reporter hadn't misquoted Dr. Hanna, why then everything was hunky-dory.

I remember one day about ten years ago when I was assistant to the New York *Herald Tribune*'s science editor and on the carpet for a front-page story in the paper that I hadn't even written. It had been written, in fact, by Earl Ubell, the science editor of the paper (and now news director of WNBC-TV in New York).

Ubell had earned a bachelor's degree in science at the City College of New York in the 1940s while working as a desk secretary to the managing editor at the *Herald Tribune* and by the early 1950s he had taken over the newspaper's science coverage. In the next ten years, this enfant terrible who couldn't be given so much as a bottle of whiskey at Christmas, and had the enthusiasm for science writing that one associates with the kid stringer for a Boston daily who's suddenly asked to cover the Red Sox or the Bruins for a week, terrorized public relations men, doctors and, most important of all, the editors of the *Herald Tribune*.

Partly because of his enormous energy, partly because of a showman's flair for dramatizing science and medicine, and partly because he did his homework with the care he'd learned in the CCNY physics laboratories, Ubell browbeat the *Tribune* editors to the point where, if the foreign desk had a story from the Soviet Union about the surgical creation of a two-headed dog that could bite a pair of mailmen simultaneously, they dared not stick it in the newspaper without clearing the matter with the science editor, Ubell, or his assistant.

As a corollary to this healthy restraint exercised by Ubell upon the generally irresponsible disposition of city and national news editors, who feel that if a science story is about sex or booze or pot or dogs or cats it can't be all bad, Ubell could also inveigle them into featuring articles by him about which they had visceral misgivings. Such a story, which led off, "There is dreadful news about breast cancer," covered the entire width of the front page of the *Herald Tribune* one day in 1964. As usual, Ubell's byline on the article indicated that it had been meticulously researched. The facts and figures showing that radical mastectomy followed by irradiation of the chest and adjacent tissues did not affect survival of the female patients, came from a respected institution, Johns Hopkins University. (The content of the article was identical with that of the 1974 preliminary findings of the NCI breast cancer task force.)

When the storm broke the morning the story appeared, Ubell was nowhere to be found. He wasn't hiding; he was probably returning from a well-paid lecture. Some women called in, sobbing. Some husbands whose wives had recently had the operation and the radiation arrived at the *Tribune* city room in person. As Ubell's assistant, it was my job to greet these visitors and try to calm them down. Mostly, I spent my time denying that I was Ubell, commiserating with them, and worrying about whether they had a pistol in their pocket. In the aftermath of recriminations at the newspaper, there appeared to be two schools of thought, and the depth of cerebration involved should provide a fair idea of the competence of most newspaper editors to cope with any event or information more sophisticated than a train-wreck. One school of thought at the *Herald Tribune* said that the article was okay but should not have been run atop page one. The other school thought that the positioning of the story was all right but that the lead sentence was a little gloomy.

Television editors handling science news have an additional handicap compared to newspaper types. As well as asking whether the story will be of interest to millions of viewers and whether it is capable of being encapsulated in 90 seconds or less, they must also ask whether it has "visual impact"—can you show on the little screen what the doctor, astronomer, psychologist, oceanographer is doing? Add to that the ancillary question: How much will it cost to draw a picture or make a model to show what he or she is doing? This being the case, it is easy to see why space and underwater ventures in science are more adequately covered by video than are flatworm-learning stories or stars that have only been "observed" by their radio emissions.

That the science menu should be limited by the susceptibility of the entree to photography is comprehensible if not always for-givable. However, when acupuncture takes precedence over im-munology because the former is easily shown and the latter is not, one begins to sense the camera usurping editorial function.

There is, of course, no proof that, in a given instance, the abil-ity of the video camera to encompass certain data and not others influences the news coverage. Frank Field, the optometrist weathercaster of New York's NBC station, has, among other TV science editors, made herculean efforts to show how science works and has a half-hour syndicated program in which he com-bined a spontaneous but unobtrusive interviewing technique with whatever visuals he could cajole the scientist into supply-ing. Sometimes the art or microscopic movies or models were fascinating, sometimes they were dull, but Field was given the time and hence gave his interviewed subject time to explain the matter at hand, invariably coming in with an elucidating ques-tion when the interviewee wandered into poppy fields of jargon.

One Saturday evening Field's home station took advantage of his absence to cover and air a part of a convention on acupuncture. This was in October 1974 when fast-buck operators were already moving in on the publicity that had been accorded the Chinese needling technique as a result of renewed coverage of that country so long off limits to Americans. That evening, Channel 4 New York told us about a new use for acupuncture in people who were obese and wanted to stop overeating or were alcoholic and wanted to stop drinking or, as I recall, were just plain depressed. (I must rely on memory here because NBC News says it is unable to supply the transcript of the broadcast for my inspection.) Next came remote footage of a doctor standing by a hospital stretcher on which reclined a comely young woman. The doctor told the viewer he could treat certain emotional problems by inserting a small pin in the patient's ear. He proceeded to demonstrate this method, using what appeared to be a version of a stapling gun of the type employed by builders and carpenters in tacking up insulation. The young woman smiled. It obviously didn't hurt and it only took a few seconds. It was all very visual. Now back to the reporter who assured us that other, unspecified doctors weren't convinced that the staple version of acupuncture was any improvement on the needle's achievement in deafness, which had been found to be nil, and that such treatment would be unlikely to replace conventional approaches to the therapy such patients needed.

Astonished that such a gimmicky piece of arrant quackery should have been given time on the air and with such a brief and colorless disclaimer at its conclusion—it would have helped at least to have seen a real psychiatrist on camera, no matter how briefly, to put this nonsense down—I wrote the news director of WNBC-TV, none other than the formidable Earl Ubell. His answer emphasized the goal of the Federal Communications Commission in achieving over-all balance in the presentation of opposing ideas on television. He also wrote to me that because the NBC segment came from a meeting devoted to the subject of acupuncture, the television editors had felt it was adequate to balance the plug for ear stapling with a general statement that there were a number of physicians who did not endorse the technique. Thus Ubell presented a picture of a scale whose balancing pans were loaded on one side or the other over a period of weeks or months, and he implied that this process and not the statements made on any single newscast were critical to public understanding.

A week after Ubell's sophisticated explanation arrived, *Newsweek*, with pictures of staple in place and stapling gun in firing position weighed the pros and cons in aiding dieters. Along with a comment from the American Medical Association that it had no scientific evidence that a staple in the ear reduced hunger, *Newsweek* quoted Dr. Robert H. Moser, the editor of the AMA's official publication, to the effect that he had heard some disquieting reports about patients who had no examination before being stapled and put on a 400-calorie diet and about a staple center that was charging $45 for a quick staple job with no follow-through. The clinician interviewed for the *Newsweek* article, a New York City internist named Josué M. Corcos, said he insisted on a thorough examination before applying staples and recommending diets and that he had his patients apply an antibiotic ointment twice daily to the stapled site to prevent infection. It was not clear just how the theory of acupuncture was involved since Dr. Corcos said he just instructed the patient to twiddle the staple a little when hunger pangs set in. He termed it "just a helpful extra for the compulsive eater." Not one of these nuances or warnings was given any attention during the NBC newscast.

But wait; for any viewers who had not sallied forth in October, November, or December to get their ears stapled and enhance their will power, WNBC-TV supplied an exposée prophylaxis in mid-January 1975. Suddenly on my television set I heard from an adjoining room Frank Field saying, "We're not against acupuncture. We're for the right for people to practice acupuncture. We're also for the right for doctors to do it." Sensing that another chunk of heavy metal was about to be slung onto the other pan of the Ubell-Federal Communications Commission scales, I dashed for the living room to grab my tape recorder. Yes, this was the night for staplers to get theirs.

Field showed us an ear staple. He said it was the "newest rage in acupuncture." He said some users lost weight, others didn't, and others had other problems. Then we saw a young woman whose ear staple had become painful after a few days. Field told us the young woman had proceeded to the office of her Brooklyn gynecologist to have him take the staple out again. The gynecologist tried but couldn't. Then she called internists. They referred her to surgeons. Surgeons said that would involve minor surgery and what she called "a large charge." Then she tried acupuncture clinics but "they wouldn't touch it because someone else had put it in." Finally, after imploring her gynecologist once more but with similar results, she went to the emergency room of a major New York hospital. There, a surgical resident found pus coming out of the staple holes. After X-raying the patient's ear to make certain just how long the staple was, he injected a local anesthetic and removed it. Judging by personal experience in the emergency rooms of New York's big voluntary hospitals, the removal cost the young woman at least as much as the insertion.

But now there came up the issue of the legality of the whole procedure. Field told us the young woman had not signed informed consent to the use of a research procedure on her body. That is required by New York State for unapproved piercing of the body for medical purposes (as opposed to aesthetic ones). The fact that the State Board of Regents had not promptly collared the offending gynecologist, who, contrary to Ubell's impression, claimed he had not been practicing acupuncture, only obesity control, horrified one of the anchormen on the WNBC-TV news show. He remonstrated with Field about the state's inaction. But then, the new anchorman, Tom Snyder, had been out on the West Coast at some other station when, on that Saturday night in October, the other pan had been loaded.

The problem of balance is an old one and, even if it could be solved in a fashion satisfactory to everyone, is no adequate replacement for sound judgment. Where public fears and desires about health and beauty, cancer and heart disease, sex and procreation are involved, there would seem to be at least as great a need for the latter commodity as there is in a state or local election. Maybe more.

One solution used in medical coverage by a number of responsible daily newspapers is the roundup, in which the science reporter works up a single topic into a series of two or more long articles bringing the readers up to date in a given field. Every year the majority of medical and science writing prizes are awarded by their sponsoring organizations to the authors of such series, where there is space to present opposing points of view.

How editors may be converted to a more sophisticated, and less gee-whiz attitude toward science stories I leave to the National Association of Science Writers, which has made sporadic efforts in that direction. In all likelihood, nothing can be done about the obdurate atavism of the news industry.

My recommendation for readers who feel short-changed in keeping abreast of scientific developments is not to write to editors or congressmen, which will do no earthly good, but instead to take a weekly course of immunization by subscribing to the British publication *The New Scientist* and supplementing that with a booster that can be had in most good public libraries, the "News and Comment" section of *Science*, the weekly publication mentioned earlier in these pages. Complete immunity to the trivia and exaggeration that masquerades as science in many quarters may take a year or more of such reading to achieve. It's probably the only protection available, though.

APPENDIX 1

Report of Summerlin Peer Review Committee

PRESENTED TO DR. LEWIS THOMAS, PRESIDENT
MEMORIAL SLOAN-KETTERING CANCER CENTER

MAY 17, 1974

Contents of the Report

I. SUMMARY OF FINDINGS

1. By his admission, first to Drs. Lloyd J. Old and Robert A. Good on March 26, 1974, and subsequently to the Peer Review Committee on May 10, 1974, Dr. William T. Summerlin early on the morning of March 26 used a pen to darken the site where the skin had previously been grafted on each of two mice which he was to exhibit to Dr. Good that morning.

2. Although a few mice apparently bearing successful allografts or xenografts of skin and representing work done by Dr. Summerlin at Minnesota had been available for inspection there and were exhibited at Sloan-Kettering Institute before Dr. Summerlin transferred to this Institute, the only such mouse available to the committee at the time of their inquiry was the so-called Old Man. This mouse, which has been continuously represented by Dr. Summerlin as an example of a permanently successful skin graft crossing the histocompatibility barrier, is now proved to be a hybrid rather than an inbred mouse, implying that the graft was accepted for well-recognized genetic reasons. It remains a matter of conjecture how this mistake came about, and whether the other ostensibly successful transplants of Dr. Summerlin's may similarly have explanations not based on crossing histocompatibility barriers.

3. Dr. Summerlin, by his admission to the committee, incorrectly and repeatedly exhibited or reported on certain rabbits as each having had two human corneal transplants, one unsuccessful from a fresh cornea and the other successful from a cultured cornea, whereas, in fact, only one cornea had been transplanted to each rabbit and all were unsuccessful. He admitted that he did not know, nor was he in a position to know, which rabbit was which, and that he only assumed what procedures had been carried out on the rabbits he exhibited. This grossly misleading assumption as totally unwarrantable from the beginning, and even more so after the discrepancy had been pointed out to him. The committee, however, recognizes that the prolonged preservation of human corneas in culture may be of significant value.

4. The more recent transplantations of adrenals in C3H mice did not show as good results as were reported in the Minnesota experiments. At best the results with the adrenal and the parathyroid transplants at Sloan-Kettering were equivocal; consequently little weight was given by the committee to these observations, as compared with the more serious questions raised by the presentations of the mouse skin grafts and of the human corneal transplants to rabbits.

5. The committee recognizes a number of promising indications from the use of cultured human skin, suggesting that this may be a suitable area for renewed evaluation of the method.

6. Some of the broader aspects of this inquiry are dealt with in the section General Considerations.

II. RECOMMENDATIONS

In reviewing these findings, the committee members believe that some actions of Dr. Summerlin over a considerable period of time were not those of a responsible scientist. It is recommended that Dr. Summerlin be offered a medical leave of absence to alleviate his situation, which may have been exacerbated by pressure of the many obligations which he voluntarily undertook. For whatever reason, he has been led to irresponsible conduct that is incompatible with discharge of his responsibilities in the scientific community.

It is the opinion of the committee that it is in the best interests of both Dr. Summerlin and of Sloan-Kettering Institute that his association with the Institute be terminated. A main factor in deciding the date of this termination should be whether Dr. Summerlin assents to the need for medical leave of absence expressly for the reasons set forth in this report.

III. INTRODUCTION

On March 26, 1974, Dr. William T. Summerlin, Member of the Sloan-Kettering Institute, admitted to Dr. Robert A. Good and Dr. Lloyd J. Old, President and Director, and Vice-President and Associate Director of the Institute, respectively, that, as reported to them by members of his laboratory group, he had used his pen to darken the skin transplant area of two mice before showing them to Dr. Good early that morning. This promptly led to his temporary suspension from all administrative and scientific activities in the Institute. On April 5, Dr. Good requested a group of senior scientists to serve on a peer review committee to review the validity of Dr. Summerlin's scientific activities and together with Dr. Old met at that time with a majority of the group. Dr. Good's appointment of the committee and his charge to it were reaffirmed formally in his letter of May 3 to the chairman of the committee. The committee was requested to report to the President of Memorial Sloan-Kettering Cancer Center, Dr. Lewis Thomas.

After much of the inquiry by the committee had taken place and before it had met with Dr. Summerlin, he raised an objection to Dr. John Hadden's membership on the committee. Without agreeing to the merit of the objection, the committee accepted Dr. Hadden's offer to withdraw from the committee. The remainder of the committee wishes to express its appreciation for his valuable service while a member of the committee.

While various aspects of Dr. Summerlin's scientific activities were to come under scrutiny of the committee, it was decided early to concentrate upon the questionable results or apparent misrepresentations involved in the mouse skin grafting and the corneal grafts in rabbits.

The committee sought a number of affidavits and written statements pertinent to its inquiry. In addition interviews were held with 17 individuals including Dr. Summerlin, who appeared before the committee for approximately 8 hours. Numerous telephone calls to scientists at the University of Minnesota and other parts of the country provided other essential information.

The committee has attempted to pursue all leads to information which it believed might contribute to the determination of the truth in each important aspect of its review. While the committee did concern itself with the scientific basis of enhanced transplantability of tissues and organs placed in culture, it interpreted its primary task as being to decide whether, and to what extent, Dr. Summerlin had misrepresented findings and observations in regard to this subject.

IV. MICE RECEIVING ALLOGRAFTS OR XENOGRAFTS OF SKIN

To review in detail all the events related to this work is not feasible. This report is focused on those carefully selected aspects of it which were of the most value in enabling the committee to reach its conclusions. Further evidence is available and could be subjected to similar detailed scrutiny; but the committee is satisfied that the general import of this additional material would serve to strengthen its present conclusions.

(1) The facts relating to March 26, 1974, which precipitated the present inquiry are not in any significant respect disputed by Dr. Summerlin and so need only be outlined here. (These details are a matter of record.)

Dr. Summerlin stated to the committee on May 10 that while conveying a selection of his mice to a meeting requested by Dr. Good, which took place around 7:00 A.M., he "touched up" or blackened the grafted areas on two white mice. The cages were conveyed back to Dr. Summerlin's animal room by him about an hour later. The mice had been only cursorily inspected by Dr. Good, who was concerned at this meeting primarily with a manuscript which he proposed should be published by Drs. Ninnemann, Good and Summerlin concerning the negative results of the skin culture method in the hands of Dr. Ninnemann, a Fellow of Dr. Good's working in Dr. Summerlin's laboratory. Some time after 9:00 A.M., a Senior Laboratory Assistant, James Martin, in returning the cages to their places, noted that the appearance of the supposed black grafts on two white mice was unfamiliar. On applying alcohol, he discovered black material that could be washed away. The matter was brought to the attention of a Senior Research Technician, William Walter, then of Dr. O'Neill, a Visiting Research Fellow, and also of Dr. Raaf, a Research Fellow. Dr. Raaf recalled having been shown these two mice by Dr. Summerlin earlier in the day, who represented them to Dr. Raaf as successful transplants. Dr. Raaf informed Drs. Old and Good of the apparent misrepresentation.

In regard to why a report was not first made to Dr. Summerlin himself, the committee perceived especially from evidence of Dr. O'Neill, Dr. Raaf and Dr. Ninnemann that an atmosphere of incredulity, frustration and disillusion had developed among the professional personnel in Dr. Summerlin's laboratory group; the committee believes that in these circumstances a direct report to Drs. Good and Old was understandable and proper, and was made solely from the correct and over-riding motive or arriving at the truth of the matter in the most direct way possible.

Around noon, Dr. Summerlin met with Drs. Good and Old, and confirmed he had blackened the mice, whereupon Dr. Good temporarily suspended Dr. Summerlin from all his duties pending further inquiry.

As was the case when Dr. Summerlin was originally confronted by Drs. Good and Old, Dr. Summerlin before the committee on May 10 again expressed himself unable to account for this action in blackening the mice.

(2) It is not in dispute that in Dr. Summerlin's quarters the only mouse obviously carrying a fully accepted skin allograft which had been retained over a prolonged period, since Dr. Summerlin's arrival at MSKCC in March 1973, was one nicknamed "The Old Man." Dr. Summerlin explained to us on May 10 that he knew it to be a female, but the name had stuck because it originally was kept together with cages of males (which Dr. Summerlin usually worked with in preference to females) that were collectively referred to as "The Old Men."

After the blackening episode, Dr. Good asked Dr. Boyse to test this mouse to decide whether it might be an F_1 hybrid, which could explain the acceptance of white (albino) skin by an agouti (wild-type speckled coat) recipient solely on a well-known genetic basis. By inspection alone, a C3H mouse cannot be distinguished from a hybrid between the C3H and A mouse strains.

Among the experimental goals suggested to Dr. Summerlin by Dr. Good when Dr. Summerlin first arrived at Minnesota was the successful transfer of A strain (albino) mouse skin to C3H strain (agouti) mouse recipients, the colour combination stated above. The "Old Man" had been grafted on 11/22/1971, according to the label on the cage. Tests in the laboratory of Dr. Boyse, carried out on blood taken from this mouse on 4/3/74, reveal it to be a hybrid (bio-chemical test for the enzyme glucosephosphate isomerase) and to give the H-2 (blood group) reactions of hybrid between C3H and A. We conclude that this one available impressive case of skin graft acceptance has the well-established explanation of genetic compatibility. Hybrids of C3H and A were available at Minnesota at the time "The Old Man" was grafted (statement of Dr. Biggar; and animal records from Minnesota).

The committee found it difficult to credit that Dr. Summerlin could have been continuously ignorant of this elementary possibility, which became ever more critical as this mouse assumed the role of a single exceptional success, or that he remained unaware that simple tests by any of several colleagues could immediately have settled the matter.

(3) Concerning the overall success of the mouse skin allograft program initiated by Dr. Summerlin at Minnesota in 1971 on Dr. Good's advice, Dr. Summerlin has written the following:

". . . . . work . . . . with mice, using homologous (allogeneic) skin grafts from standard cultures, shows that such foreign grafts are routinely accepted without rejection" (p. 2, Research grant application dated 5/31/73: Dr. Summerlin principal investigator).

This conflicts with: "In numerous adult mouse whole skin culture homografting experiments performed thus far, it appears that such grafts take without rejection if the grafting is carried out after 7–10 days in culture. These results were confirmed in 50% of such animals which were followed for up to five months. As stated previously, these grafts were transplanted across major well-defined histocompatibility barriers in mouse strains C57B1/6,DBA/2 and A/J" (Damon Runyon

Research grant application dated May 1, 1973/June 15, 1973; Dr. Summerlin principal investigator).

No data in scientific form have ever been presented for either of these alternative statements, which parallel published statements appearing in two abstracts of papers presented at meetings in 1973. One or two mice bearing grafts of a different color is all that any witness appears to have seen at any one time. This lack of properly organized and analyzable data is one of the reasons why Dr. Good in the latter part of Nov. 1973 insisted on withdrawing a paper written by Drs. Summerlin, Stutman and Good, previously submitted to the Journal of Experimental Medicine. Table 1 of this manuscript purports to show percentage acceptances of mouse skin allografts, but these do not correspond with the absolute numbers of mice cited in the same table. Dr. Summerlin at that time proffered the explanation that the percentages column referred to overall results, inclusive of data previous to that on which the table was founded. When pressed on this point before the committee on May 10, Dr. Summerlin produced a sheet of unidentified numbers that failed to clarify the issue. Asked why many of the successfully grafted recipients claimed were not retained for display and observation, Dr. Summerlin gave the astonishing reply that they were sacrificed at intervals to provide serum to be stored for H-2 antibody tests at a later date. It is scarcely conceivable that Dr. Summerlin could have believed, in such immunologically sophisticated surroundings as Dr. Good's group at Minnesota, that it is necessary to kill a mouse to obtain serum. Asked then to state what criteria he applied to the more than 100 grafted mice in order to calculate the "% grafts accepted" figures for the Journal of Experimental Medicine manuscript, which must also have formed the basis for all his public statements on the subject, Dr. Summerlin gave no coherent reply, and implied that even a few days of prolonged graft survival under ill-defined conditions might be considered "success."

Because of their epoch-making implications, Dr. Summerlin's haziness in recollecting the success-rates with xenografts of guinea pig and pig skin to mice is astonishing. Although only "prolonged acceptance" was ever claimed for these xenografts, Dr. Summerlin was unclear as to how many grafts of this kind from culture were attempted, or succeeded, and if so for how long. In answer to a question from the committee Dr. Summerlin stated that no immunosuppressive treatment of recipient mice was used to facilitate the acceptance of allografts or xenografts. No opportunity now arises for the testing of mice with long-accepted xenografts, such as the mouse bearing an apparently healthy guinea pig skin graft which several people saw, because no such mice have survived.

Against numerous reports of failure to repeat his work on allografts of cultured mouse skin from highly authoritative sources, Dr. Summerlin cites a number of successes or promising results. None of these can stand critical evaluation at the present time. For example, Dr. Prunieras, a Visiting Investigator in Dr. Summerlin's laboratory, submitted to Dr. Wachtel (an expert in skin grafting who works in Dr. Boyse's group) two mice which he considered might represent successful acceptance of cultured DBA/2 mouse skin on C57B1 mouse recipients. But Dr. Wachtel was unable to find definite evidence of surviving DBA/2 skin. This emphasizes the pitfalls in evaluating the significance of white or pale hair growth in the neighborhood of graft-sites, which may represent no more than traumatic side-effects of graft-rejection and healing. Again, a black graft may lose many of its pigment cells in culture, and when transplanted to an identical black mouse may therefore closely simulate acceptance of a white allograft by a black mouse.

In the light of Dr. Summerlin's failure to enunciate to the committee even approximate criteria adopted for a successful graft, and of his continued failure to produce adequate tabulations and criteria relating to the mouse skin grafting program, his written and verbal statements of the kind made in the grant applications cited above must be discounted.

Thus while not intending to deny the possibility of such a phenomenon, nor the extreme importance of ascertaining whether it can be accomplished, the committee is of the opinion that there exists at the present time no definitive evidence from any source that any mouse has ever obviously accepted an H-2-incompatible skin graft, or a skin xenograft, permanently or for a prolonged period, as a consequence solely of previous maintenance of the prospective graft in culture. In the circumstances now prevailing the committee has no authenticated evidence on which to form a judgement on the manner in which the few instances of mice bearing or purporting to bear successful skin allografts or skin xenografts, exhibited in the past by Dr. Summerlin, were actually achieved.

Fellow investigators are justified in assuming that pronouncements of new observations by other scientists are made on the basis of adequate data, systematically obtained, recorded, and interpreted, according to accepted standards of investigation; since this is evidently not the case with Dr. Summerlin's experiments with mice it is the opinion of the committee that he has propagated misconceptions concerning the nature and scope of his work in this area.

V. CORNEAL GRAFTS

Minnesota Experience

The corneal grafting in question was started at the University of Minnesota during the summer of 1972 when Dr. George E. Miller, then a resident in Opthalmology, entered into collaboration with Dr. Summerlin to examine the possibility of transplanting cultured corneas. During the summer and until December 1972, Dr. Miller performed the transplantation work, including animal care and maintenance, in the Department of Ophthalmology and worked with Dr. Summerlin in his laboratory maintaining the corneal cultures. The transplants at that time were of 2 types:

1. Intralamellar corneal transplants in which a piece of cultured or noncultured cornea was placed in a pocket retro-orbitally to the limbus (a nonprivileged site immunologically) in order to evaluate the inflammatory reaction descriptive of an immunologic reaction to the grafted material. Donor grafts were guinea pig, human, chicken and rabbit. Each recipient rabbit received only a single graft.

2. Centrally placed keratoplasty transplants were of 4–5 mm size. Again only one eye of a rabbit recipient was operated upon (no limbus to limbus penetrating transplants were performed as this is technically impossible, according to Dr. Doughman, in the rabbit because the anterior chamber is thus compromised and glaucoma results).

Corneal xenografts from guinea pig and human donors were unsuccessful by both techniques if the criterion used was survival for greater than 40 days. In a small series of approximately 10 animals each, xenografts from chickens and allografts from rabbits showed prolonged survival and reduced immunogenicity in some but not all recipients. There was no permanent acceptance of any corneal xenografts; specifically none of the human xenografts survived longer than 40 days.

During the course of these experiments it was found that corneas could be preserved in culture for relatively long periods and subsequently transplanted successfully, a finding of considerable significance in its application to future human corneal preservation and allografting.

In December of 1972 the collaboration between Dr. Summerlin and the ophthalmologists in Minnesota was dissolved over a dispute about priority of authorship. However, prior to his talk at the American Society of Clinical Investigation in May 1973, Dr. Summerlin was provided with data on 35 mm slides showing some temporary acceptance (up to 40 days) of guinea pig and chicken corneal grafts in rabbits. Since this time the work with rabbit allografts and xenografts (chicken, not human) has continued in Minnesota under the auspices of Drs. Donald Doughman and John E. Harris. There was no further submission of detailed experimental results to Dr. Summerlin, but he was informed subsequently by Dr. Doughman that the original results could not be repeated although the experiments were not totally unsuccessful.

Despite these spotty results, Dr. Summerlin has made the following reports based on the Minnesota experience:

1. March 30, 1973—Written statement to the press at the American Cancer Society Science Writers Seminar: "We have since attempted to extend this work to other organ systems and find that whole cornea from a number of species, human included, functions quite normally during the culture process and is transplanted without rejection (xenogenically and allogenically) into rabbit-eye recipients."

2. *J. Clin. Invest.*, 52:83a, 1973, (Abstract No. 307), for an address to the American Society of Clinical Investigation in May 1973: "Allotransplants and xenotransplants of cornea near limbus are accepted and have exhibited good function for six months. Control allogenic and xenogenic grafts placed near the limbus are regularly rejected within two weeks."

3. Stated in a manuscript in preparation, "The organ cultured cornea: an *in vivo* assessment of antigenicity," by William T. Summerlin, Robert A. Good, George E. Miller and John E. Harris:

> "All intralamellar corneal transplants that were cultured beyond three weeks took without usual evidence of rejection. Such completely accepted xenografts at the limbus have been followed now for more than six months without signs of rejection. By contrast, control, noncultured grafts have been promptly rejected by the 14th day. Slit lamp examination of the corneas grafted from culture shows complete clarity in contrast to the opacity of the rejected control grafts."

Dr. Miller was consulted by telephone concerning this manuscript which was apparently based upon his work but written by Dr. Summerlin. He indicated no prior knowledge of this paper and stated that the results could not have been his since *all* cultured intralamellar xenografts according to his protocol meant guinea pig, chicken, and human. Although he had partial and temporary success with guinea pig and chicken corneal grafts, there was no successful xenograft of human corneas at Minnesota.

New York Experience

All of the corneal grafting at Sloan-Kettering was performed by Dr. Peter Laino, an ophthalmologist at New York Hospital, or by one of his residents, Dr. Bartley Mondino. Their association with Dr. Summerlin began in approximately May 1973 after Dr. H. Randolph Guthrie had approached Dr. Laino about the work Dr. Summerlin was doing and a meeting was arranged with Dr. Summerlin. Dr. Summerlin outlined the corneal grafting project already in progress at the University of Minnesota and indicated that he would like to disassociate himself from the Minnesota project and instead work in collaboration with Dr. Laino at Sloan-Kettering. Protocols were developed in which design Dr. Summerlin participated. Fresh human cadaver corneas were obtained by Dr. Laino from the New York Eye Bank and transplanted into rabbits provided by Dr. Summerlin. Although one of the protocols called for paired fresh and cultured corneas from the same cadaver to be transplanted to both eyes of a rabbit recipient, this protocol was never implemented and in all experiments only one eye received a transplant, the other serving as an unoperated control.

The project started in June 1973 with all the work being done in the Kettering Laboratory. During June, July and August Dr. Laino worked alone because Dr. Mondino was away during those months. Most of the work during those early months was devoted to learning techniques of rabbit corneal transplantation and culturing corneas. Dr. Mondino returned in September and performed much of the work thereafter. No cultured corneas were transplanted until the end of September or early October 1973. Drs. Laino and Mondino kept all their records at New York Hospital and coded the animal cages with numbers; Dr. Summerlin did not have access to the records nor did he know the code.

It was found that the human corneas were very well preserved in culture and that there was good morphological evidence of viability for up to six months; Dr. Laino and Dr. Mondino were very pleased that the corneas were so well preserved *in vitro* and they are preparing a report on this aspect of the work for publication.

Dr. Laino's letter of February 25, 1974, to Dr. Summerlin, stated that "a total of about 20 rabbits have been grafted with human donor material that was first passed through tissue culture. It appears that no appreciable difference in acceptance or rejection time occurs when these eyes are compared to others grafted directly into recipients without having first been passed through tissue culture. They both fail about the same time." Dr. Mondino also told the committee that there was no difference in the survival of fresh and cultured human cornea grafts and that all were uniformly rejected at about the same time. Their attempts to transplant human corneas were abandoned in late December 1973 because of the lack of success.

Dr. Laino and Dr. Mondino had almost no communication with Dr. Summerlin during the entire period. Dr. Laino does recall that, in mid-October 1973, he and Dr. Mondino showed Dr. Summerlin one or two rabbits which had received a human corneal graft in only one eye. They both deny that they ever led Dr. Summerlin to believe that any of the human corneal xenografts were successful or that any of the rabbits had received bilateral grafts. Although Dr. Summerlin admitted that he was never told by Dr. Laino and Dr. Mondino that any of their rabbits had received bilateral transplants (one fresh and one cultured human cornea), he said he was under the impression that this was the case since one of the original protocols drawn up by himself and Dr. Laino called for paired corneal transplants using both eyes from the same cadaver donor. Dr. Summerlin in fact stated that he was not aware that this protocol had never been implemented until April 22, 1974, when he was specifically told by Dr. Laino that none of the rabbits had received transplants in both eyes.

On the other hand, Drs. Good, Raaf and Ninnemann each recalls being specifically told by Dr. Summerlin in September 1973 or earlier that at least some of the rabbits had received grafts in both eyes, one of cultured and one of fresh cornea, and that only the cultured corneas had taken successfully. They were each shown rabbits by Dr. Summerlin which were alleged to have cultured human corneal grafts in place on the unoperated eye; they all expressed amazement since the eye looked perfectly normal and there was no evidence of suture lines.

Dr. Summerlin brought two rabbits to the Board of Scientific Consultants meeting on October 4, 1973, which he had told Dr. Good had both eyes grafted with human corneas with the normal appearing eye being the recipient of a cultured graft. Dr. Good then so presented these rabbits to the Board of Scientific Consultants on the basis of what Dr. Summerlin had told him. Dr. Good stressed to the review committee that at that time he had never met Dr. Laino or Dr. Mondino, and he was entirely dependent on Dr. Summerlin's representation of their work. Dr. Good further stated that he was unaware that none of the rabbits had received bilateral transplants until after Dr. Summerlin was suspended in late March 1974.

Following the October 4, 1973, Board of Scientific Consultants meeting at which Drs. Raaf and Ninnemann were present, according to their statements they checked with Dr. Mondino to see if any of the rabbits had been grafted on both eyes. When told by Dr. Mondino that this was not the case, they so informed Dr. Summerlin. Dr. Summerlin told the Committee that he does not recall being so informed, but he admitted that without checking further he subsequently presented rabbits on at least 6 separate occasions during which he claimed that the normal appearing (unoperated) eye had received a cultured human corneal graft:

> October 14 and 15, 1973—National Cancer Institute Site Visit;
> October 19, 1973—American Cancer Society Site Visit (Dr. Amos and Dr. Milgrom);
> November 3, 1973—Dr. Good's internal review of Dr. Summerlin's program;
> November 16, 1973—Visit of Representative Paul Rogers;
> January 7, 1974—National Cancer Institute Site Visit by Dr. Billingham;
> January 7, 1974—Memorial Sloan-Kettering Cancer Center Combined Staff Conference.

In addition, articles appeared in the March 15, 1974, issue of *Medical World News* and the April 1974 issue of *Clinical Trends* in each of which there was a photograph showing both eyes of a rabbit, one of which is cloudy and said in the caption to represent a noncultured human corneal graft undergoing rejection 30 days after the implant. Prior to publication of the article, Dr. Laino was called by Mr. Ames of *Medical World News*, and he specifically denied that this could have been one of his rabbits since he had never operated on both eyes and had no successful human cultured corneal grafts. Dr. Laino advised Mr. Ames to call Dr. Summerlin to find out whose rabbit was portrayed in the photograph. Dr. Summerlin talked to Mr. Ames of *Medical World News* on several occasions and to Dr. Jean Watson of *Clinical Trends* prior to the appearance of these articles; he made several corrections and approved the final versions of the texts of these articles as they appeared in print. Although Dr. Summerlin stated that in neither instance was the rabbit photograph and caption referred to above submitted to him for final approval (this was confirmed by Dr. Watson and Mr. Ames who said it was not their policy to furnish final proofs of such photographs), the photograph in *Clinical Trends* was obtained by Ms. Phyllis Shaw from Dr. Summerlin himself and transmitted to Dr. Watson for her use. Dr. Summerlin wrote Dr. Howard Cohn of *Medical World News* on April 23, 1974, "Though I thoroughly reviewed this article with your staff prior to publication, regrettably I was not consulted about the final photo caption." In this letter, he also told Dr. Cohn that the caption was erroneous since, after checking with Dr. Laino, he realized that the rabbit photographed had only received one corneal graft.

There is no dispute that Dr. Summerlin raised no objection to the following statement in the text of the *Clinical Trends* article, "They are implanting in rabbit eyes human corneas that have been immersed in organ culture medium for more than a month. Transplants not only take, but they remain clear for up to several months. Somehow during their long stay in the culture medium, the corneas have retained their viability and lost some of their immunogenicity." According to Dr. Watson, Dr. Summerlin was sent the final version of this article on March 29, 1974, which included this statement and returned it to Dr. Watson on April 1, 1974, with his approval for publication.

Committee's Appraisal of Dr. Summerlin's Representation of Work on Rabbits Receiving Human Corneal Transplants.

The question whether deliberate misrepresentation was involved in this work can be viewed from the standpoint of whether it was possible under the circumstances for anyone in Dr. Summerlin's position to have mistakenly supposed a rabbit to have received a corneal graft to each eye rather than to only one. Dr. Summerlin states he believed the protocol called for each rabbit to receive a fresh cornea in one eye, and a cultured cornea from the same donor in the other eye. There would in this event be a period during which each rabbit carried only one corneal graft while the other was being cultured. There could be no assurance that the second graft would actually be applied later because it might be lost by infection of the culture or by accident or any other fortuitous circumstances; or the operation might be postponed or cancelled for reasons unknown to Dr. Summerlin. Therefore it was manifestly impossible for anyone to deduce whether the second eye of any rabbit had been operated upon, except by observing operative trauma to the second eye or by consulting the records. In fact, no rabbit was doubly grafted, so there never was any rabbit with signs of operation on the second eye. Neither could the records have been consulted, because Dr. Laino kept the records in his possession and these were coded—a usual precaution to preserve objectivity in observation. And had the records been available to Dr. Summerlin, they would have disclosed exclusively single grafting, i.e., one corneal graft per rabbit. There was no possibility, therefore, of mistaking a singly grafted rabbit for a doubly grafted rabbit, because whatever Dr. Summerlin may have thought the protocol called for, there was never any indication of any kind, from any rabbit itself or from the records, that the second operation supposed to be called for had been carried out. Before the Committee, Dr. Summerlin gave no rational explanation of how anyone could conclude that any particular rabbit had been doubly grafted. Dr. Summerlin could not suggest any way in which Dr. Good's misapprehension that some rabbits had been doubly grafted could have come about other than through Dr. Summerlin himself.

Dr. Summerlin now states (May 10, 1974) that he was uncertain whether any rabbits had in fact been doubly grafted but that he had great difficulty in reaching Dr. Laino or Dr. Mondino to verify this. This is an unacceptable justification of how the rabbits could be mistaken by him as having been doubly grafted, and were so misrepresented by Dr. Summerlin over many months. It is undeniable that, in a matter as vital and urgent as the protocol applied to these rabbits, which were exhibited as evidence of a triumphal crossing of transplantation barriers, the necessary information could have been obtained within a day or so at the longest, either personally or by note-of-hand, or by a call to the private residence of Dr. Laino or Dr. Mondino, or by some other means of communication. The only possible conclusion is that Dr. Summerlin was responsible for initiating and perpetuating a profound and serious misrepresentation about the results of transplanting cultured human corneas to rabbits.

VI. HUMAN SKIN GRAFTS

Before coming to Memorial Sloan-Kettering Cancer Center, Dr. Summerlin had reported a number of successful allogenic cultured skin grafts. At least one of these cases is now available for biopsy three years after the original transplant of female skin. Confirmatory evidence of prolonged survival of cultured allogeneic human skin grafts was given by Dr. Karasek in his discussion of Dr. Summerlin's paper given at the American Society of Clinical Investigation in May 1973.

During his time at Memorial Hospital Dr. Summerlin has done four clinical transplants of cultured allogeneic skin. One more was done by his fellow, Dr. Safai, immediately after Dr. Summerlin's suspension. Dr. Summerlin's technique has included the use of skin applied as a dressing, in addition to the actual skin graft itself.

The first patient was an alcoholic with a large traumatic ulcer. This was covered by four small grafts of cadaver skin, fresh, and 3 weeks, 5 weeks, or 8 weeks in culture. The fresh skin and the three-week culture skin were rejected but the other two were apparently doing well at 21 days when the patient left the hospital. He disappeared, refused to come back for clinic appointments and has so far not been seen since his discharge. He is now in an alcoholic home in Chester, New York, and the nurse there reports that his wound is completely healed. Whether this has healed with a retention of the five-week and eight-week cultured graft, or whether it has healed-in with his own epithelium is not known.

The second patient had psoriasis and an x-ray ulcer of his right ankle. This wound was prepared with fresh allogeneic skin dressings and then grafted with cultured human cadaver skin. This first became infected and was lost. A second graft was applied on the 12th of October 1973 and appeared to take well. This was approximately a 3 by 5 cm. graft and at day 19 still appeared to be in good condition. At that time, the 31st of October, the patient left for Germany. This graft apparently remained on until some time in December, at which time it is said by his doctor to have "dissolved into the bandage." According to his doctor he was regrafted again in January and again in March with skin sent by Dr. Summerlin, neither graft being retained. Whether these grafts were of cultured skin or of fresh allogeneic skin intended to stimulate wound healing is not clear at the moment.

The third patient had benign hypergammaglobulinemia and hyperviscosity and an ulcer as a result of stasis. A graft of her own skin had failed and she was grafted with allogeneic skin from culture. It remained on her wound in apparently good condition for at least 41 days as seen by independent observers and 56 days according to the notes when she was seen by Dr. Summerlin. Some time between the 56th and 70th day, when she was again seen by Dr. Summerlin, the graft had been lost and the ulcer was as bad as ever.

The fourth patient, a diabetic with lymphedema and a severe stasis ulcer, was grafted with human cultured skin but the graft became infected and was lost.

The fifth patient is a black male whose ulcer was due to frostbite which caused loss of most of his foot. This was grafted on March 28, 1974, by Dr. Safai with cultured allogeneic skin. The cultured skin graft is still in good condition with the exception of a small patch at the lower edge which has become infected and ulcerated, but otherwise the graft seems to be in good condition on the 40th day. It has been biopsied frequently by Dr. Safai, but this material has not yet been reviewed.

Thus in four of these five patients there appeared to be an increase in the time during which the graft persisted despite an underlying impairment of circulation which militated against graft survival. In the two persisting grafts the possibility of a permanent take has not been ruled out.

VII. ENDOCRINE TRANSPLANTATION

A. *Adrenals*

At Minnesota and as partially reported in the abstract in the Journal of Clinical Investigation (52:83a:1973) adrenalectomized mice on distilled drinking water and regular laboratory chow did not survive in contradistinction to similarly operated and maintained mice with cultured adrenal transplants. Adrenalectomized mice with fresh adrenal transplants were like the adrenalectomized controls. The mice that were adrenalectomized and transplanted with cultured adrenals responded with steroid elevation to ACTH administration and withstood cold stress. Adrenalectomized controls or mice with fresh adrenal transplants did not survive cold stress. Not all animals, control or experimental, were stressed. Dr. Summerlin stated similar, but less dramatic, results were obtained in New York. Despite the fact that C3H mice were used because they have no accessory adrenals, about 10/160 control animals in Minnesota and 10/40 control animals in New York survived. This makes evaluation of survival with transplants more difficult. Discordant information was provided by Dr. Ninnemann who said there were no differences between control and experimental groups.

B. *Parathyroids*

This work was not done at all by Dr. Summerlin but rather by Dr. John Raaf in Dr. Summerlin's laboratory. Although early, Dr. Raaf thought there was some difference between control parathyroidectomized rats and similar animals transplanted with parathyroid glands (maintenance of serum calcium levels up to 3 to 4 months), later evaluation suggested no significant difference. No experimental results

were presented in Dr. Raaf's abstract (Fed. Proc. 33:644:74) but in
the oral presentation Dr. Raaf stated that there were no significant
differences between control and transplanted (with cultured parathyroids) parathyroidectomized rats. Two of 22 cultured grafts and 8
of 13 fresh grafts lasted longer than 30 days but Dr. Raaf did not consider the results significant.

VIII. GENERAL CONSIDERATIONS

Dr. Summerlin was supplied with all the information available to
the committee which it deemed significant, so that he could have every opportunity to prepare for questions which might be put to him
when he appeared before the committee on May 10 at their invitation.

The committee finds that in several instances Dr. Summerlin did
indeed grossly mislead his colleagues in respect to experimental work
which he himself performed or was involved in. This conclusion was
reached only after thorough consideration of alternative explanations.

The committee believes that this unusual behavior of Dr. Summerlin involved at least some measure of self-deception, or some other
aberration, which hindered him from adequately gauging the import
and eventual results of his conduct. This is most evident in his misrepresentation of the corneal transplants, for ultimately the facts were
bound to be disclosed, with untoward consequences to himself. The
committee had taken this into account in formulating its recommendations.

The committee notes Dr. Summerlin's personal qualities of warmth
and enthusiasm that have engendered confidence in himself and his
findings on the part of many who have heard or met him. On the
other hand the haphazard and desultory conduct of his everyday affairs entailed constant inconveniences and more serious troubles for
others: repeated letters requesting scientific protocols unanswered, appointments and promises unkept, and juniors left without employment
or in straitened financial circumstances. The same disarray in his laboratory organization was evidently the cause of severe frustrations
among his scientific colleagues, to the point where his juniors in particular found him evasive and lost faith in him and his research. These
traits were no doubt inevitably rendered more evident and more dis-
advantageous in the broader and more demanding setting in which
he found himself placed at Memorial Sloan-Kettering Cancer Center.
The committee thinks that these aspects of his general behavior may
have been symptomatic of the frame of mind which gave rise to the
present situation.

Thorough inquiry supports the conclusion that Dr. Good did not knowingly misrepresent any of the facts connected with the Summerlin work. Any misconceptions that Dr. Good may have held were essentially acquired from Dr. Summerlin.

It would appear that the great demands made upon Dr. Good, especially after he took over the directorship, compromised his ability to personally supervise projects of Dr. Summerlin that conspicuously lacked the sound experimental planning and guidance that Dr. Good could have provided in other circumstances.

Dr. Good first developed serious misgivings about the validity of Dr. Summerlin's work in mid-November 1973 when Dr. Ninnemann, a Fellow whom Dr. Good had assigned to work in Dr. Summerlin's laboratory with the express purpose of confirming his original skin grafting experiments in mice, reported to Dr. Good that he was unable to obtain successful grafts despite use of a variety of techniques and further told Dr. Good that he suspected Dr. Summerlin was not telling the whole truth. These negative results, coupled with the inability of other well-established investigators to confirm Dr. Summerlin's findings, made Dr. Good increasingly concerned, and from November 1973 Dr. Good instituted further measures to investigate Dr. Summerlin's claims more stringently. In retrospect, even stronger measures were called for, but Dr. Good still trusted Dr. Summerlin, and he was aware of reports from several laboratories elsewhere which tended to confirm Dr. Summerlin's claims (Karasek, Balner, Prunieras).

Had the growing concern and skepticism that had entered Dr. Good's mind regarding the mouse work been directed instead to rooting out the misconceptions that had developed by late 1973 in regard to the corneal transplants, the entire matter might have been resolved at an earlier date. As it happened, the obviously culpable act of discoloration of the mice demanded this full-scale inquiry into Dr. Summerlin's activities, which might otherwise have been difficult to justify without openly impugning his character, and without which the full extent of the problem might never have been brought to light.

Widespread enthusiasm for Dr. Summerlin's work, at a time when this was generally unchallenged, led Dr. Good to appoint him Member and Laboratory Head; this appointment to such senior posts was premature, and might have been averted if it had been subject to review by senior members of the staff.

The committee feels that Dr. Good shares some of the responsibility for what many see as undue publicity surrounding Dr. Summerlin's claims, unsupported as they were by adequate authenticated data. Dr. Good was slow to respond to a suggestion of dishonesty against Dr. Summerlin at a time when several investigators were experiencing great difficulty in repeating Dr. Summerlin's experiments. However, the usual presumptions of veracity and trustworthiness on the part of co-workers would have made it quite difficult for anyone in Dr. Good's position to entertain such a notion.

The foregoing report is respectfully submitted,

Edward A. Boyse, M. D.
Staff appointment 1961

Joseph H. Burchenal, M. D.
Staff appointment 1946

Bayard D. Clarkson, M. D.
Staff appointment 1958

Martin Sonenberg, M. D., Ph. D.
Staff appointment 1949

C. Chester Stock, Ph. D., Chairman,
Summerlin Peer Review Committee
Staff appointment 1946

APPENDIX 2

Statement by William T. Summerlin, M.D.
Regarding the Sloan-Kettering Affair

MAY 28, 1974

Last Thursday evening at about eight o'clock, the attorneys for Sloan-Kettering Center read over the telephone to my attorneys a statement which they said was to be issued at a private press conference the next morning. Although my attorneys and I were not permitted to be present at the press conference, we understand that the statement was, in fact, issued to the press.

At the outset, I would like to state certain facts reported by Dr. Thomas, which I do not dispute.

First, on March 26, 1974, I darkened the skin on two out of eighteen mice which had been previously allotransplanted. This incident took place immediately prior to a private meeting with Dr. Good at seven o'clock in the morning of that day. It was not the basis for any research data or public statements. When confronted by Dr. Good at noon on the same day, I admitted this terrible incident and made no attempt to conceal it from Dr. Good or anyone else.

Secondly, for a considerable period of time prior to my suspension from SKI on March 26, 1974, and for a short period thereafter, I misunderstood and, consequently, unintentionally misrepresented one of my collaborative projects—the corneal transplant project. This project was carried out by two physicians from the Department of Ophthalmology of New York Hospital. My role in the experiment was simply to provide facilities and staff within my laboratory for the culturing of corneas and for the housing of animals. Initially, I was consulted regarding the protocols which were to be followed in these experiments, and, as finally reduced to writing, these protocols provided for both "single eye" and "double eye" transplants. In "single eye" experiments, a cultured cornea was transplanted into the right eye of a rabbit, and a fresh cornea into the right eye of a second rabbit. In "double eye" experiments, a cultured cornea was transplanted into the right eye and a fresh cornea into the left eye of the same rabbit.

Receiving erroneous information about which rabbits were operated on and observing several rabbits with clear right eyes and opaque left eyes, I assumed that the second protocol was being followed as that combination would have been impossible under the first protocol. Based on this assumption, I made several statements regarding these rabbits which I then believed were true, but which, in retrospect, have proven to be inaccurate. The physicians in charge of the experiments have admitted that these protocols were never followed. Others have claimed that they knew as early as October 8 or 9, 1973, that this was the case and further that they so informed me. Regrettably, these claims are false. In light of recent events, no one wishes more than I that the actual facts regarding the rabbits were communicated to me.

My error was not in knowingly promulgating false data, but rather in succumbing to extreme pressure placed on me by the Institute director to publicize information regarding the rabbits, information which I informed him was best known to the ophthalmologists, and to an unbearable clinical and experimental load which numbed my better judgment to consult with the ophthalmologists, rather than rely on my assumption prior to making any statements.

In fact, for a considerable period of time I have been under extreme personal and professional stress, which led to both mental and physical exhaustion. Obviously, I regret these incidents and take full responsibility for my actions, but my major regret is that, as a physician, I was unable to recognize the symptoms of acute mental exhaustion which were overtaking me prior to committing these otherwise un-thinkable acts.

The causes for this situation are two-fold, and significantly were not addressed either by Dr. Thomas or the Good Committee. First, as the youngest member of the Institute, I was charged with the re-sponsibility of heading a laboratory at the Institute, while serving as head of a clinical service at Memorial Hospital. Within my lab there were 25 separate research projects being conducted, of which the corneal study represented only an ancillary undertaking. Further, I was personally engaged in 26 collaborative efforts with scientists in ten countries. My clinical load averaged six hours out of a day that usu-ally began at 5 A.M. and, on days when I didn't sleep in the lab, ended at 6 P.M. Obviously, I was physically and mentally exhausting myself with this regimen.

Secondly, this personal pressure generated by my schedule was ag-gravated by the professional pressure which is regrettably so much a part of medical research. Time after time, I was called upon to publi-cize experimental data and to prepare applications for grants from public and private sources. There came a time in the Fall of 1973 when I had no new startling discovery, and was brutally told by Dr. Good that I was a failure in producing significant work. Thus, I was placed under extreme pressure to produce.

Because of these pressures, I became frustrated and distraught, and this culminated in the state of complete mental exhaustion which even the Center recognizes as being the only rational explanation for the incidents outlined above.

I only hope that my problem will forewarn other dedicated young researchers who could fall into the same pattern. In spite of this cur-rent difficulty, I remain committed to the medical sciences, and look forward to continuing my work.

INDEX

Aaronson, Stuart, 130
Acupuncture; 193, 194; and ear
  stapling, 194–96
Adrenal gland, 32, 35, 100
Albert Einstein College of Medicine of
  Yeshiva University, 47
Allergy, 45
Altman, Lawrence K., 88–89
American Association for the
  Advancement of Science, 87
American Burn Association, 89–90
American Cancer Society, 15, 27–28,
  29, 44, 57, 115, 119, 171; cancer
  researchers' press conferences, 28–31,
  33
American Heart Association, 117
American Legion Memorial research
  professorship, University of
  Minnesota, 16
American Medical Association (AMA),
  115, 195; *Journal* of, 21
American Society for Clinical
  Investigation, 35, 98
American Society for the Control of
  Cancer, 115
Amethopterin, 53
Anderson, Alan, Jr., 142, 143, 149, 150,
  151, 152
Anderson, M. D., Hospital and Tumor
  Institute, 19, 120, 170, 174, 181
Antibodies (immune globulins), 16, 76
Antigens, 61, 65, 75, 76, 80, 84
Associated Press, 29, 33, 86, 91, 185,
  188, 190, 191
Ataxia-telangiectasia, 62
Atomic Energy Commission, 51, 118,
  158, 168
Auerbach, Stuart, 96

Bach, Fritz, 64–65, 66
Bacteriology, 140
Baker, Carl, 120, 121, 122, 125
Balis, M. Earl, 53
Baltimore, David, 170
Baltimore *News American*, 33
Barnard, Christiaan, 14
Barr body, 25, 97–98
Bassin, Robert, 130
BCG vaccine, 149, 184, 188–91
Beattie, Edward J., Jr., 13
Bendich, Aaron, 53
Billingham, Rupert, 38, 46
Biology, 170, 171–72, 175, 177–78, 180,
  181; molecular, 122, 161, 162
Birth defects, 114

Bishop, Jerry, 28
Black, Shirley Temple, 116
Bobst, Elmer Holmes, 57
Blood: transfusion problems, 65; white
  cells, 16–18, 75–76, 79, 152
Bone marrow, 16–18, 34
Boone, Charles, 130
Borek, Ernest, 160–61
Boyse, Edward, 75, 83–84
Breast cancer, 116, 121, 168: surgery
  for, 70, 184, 186–88, 192–93; virus
  research, 158–59
Brent, Leslie, 38, 104–5
Brimble, Philip, 33
British Medical Journal, 189
Brody, Jane, 33, 34, 86–87, 96, 97, 100,
  102, 188
Bronx Veterans Administration
  Hospital, 80
Brooke Army Medical Center (burn
  center), 21, 22, 101
Brown, George, 53
Buffalo *Evening News,* 33
Burchenal, Joseph, 53, 54, 83
Burnet, MacFarlane, 61, 116
Burnet-Medawar dogma, 67, 99
Burns, skin grafts for, 21, 22, 23
Burton, Lawrence, 142, 143, 149–51, 153

Caldwell, W. E., 144
California Institute of Technology, 149
Calmette Guérin bacillus (BCG), 70
Camp, David, 17–18
Cancer, 3, 40, 113, 114; abortion by
  body's immune system, 3, 6, 18;
  animal, 152, 183; cervical (uterine),
  121, 125, 154; colon, 168; genital, 16;
  immunologic deficiency causes, 60,
  61–62, 149; induced-erysipelas
  treatment, 139–41; media
  misinformation, 168–69, 185, 186,
  188–89, 190; prostate, 116, 165;
  radiation induced, 138, 144. *See also*
  Breast Cancer; Hodgkin's disease;
  Leukemia; Tumors
Cancer Act of 1971, 119, 121, 161, 171,
  177, 185
Cancer Control, 176–77
Cancer research, 2, 15, 80, 83, 114–15,
  141, 144, 171, 187; budgeting for, 55,
  56, 58, 158–59, 163–66; and
  cancer-patient therapy, 58, 170, 172,
  181–82; conflict of interests, 130;
  cure-versus-understanding goals, 114,